# Enough, Already!

Finding Happiness Now in a World
That Wants to Sell You Perfection Later

Heather Jayne Wynn

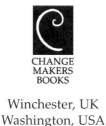

CHANGE
MAKERS
BOOKS

Winchester, UK
Washington, USA

First published by Changemakers Books, 2016
Changemakers Books is an imprint of John Hunt Publishing Ltd., Laurel House, Station Approach,
Alresford, Hants, SO24 9JH, UK
office1@jhpbooks.net
www.johnhuntpublishing.com
www.changemakers-books.com

For distributor details and how to order please visit the 'Ordering' section on our website.

ISBN: 978 1 78535 308 6
Library of Congress Control Number: 2016935417

A CIP catalogue record for this book is available from the British Library.

Design: Lee Nash


Printed in the USA by Edwards Brothers Malloy

We operate a distinctive and ethical publishing philosophy in all
areas of our business, from our global network of authors to
production and worldwide distribution.

# Enough, Already!

Finding Happiness Now in a World
That Wants to Sell You Perfection Later

# CONTENTS

# Acknowledgments

My husband, Paul, deserves a solid gold medal (but I know he'd be more than happy with new golf clubs) for seeing this journey through with me. 'Thank you' doesn't quite cover it, for he is, and always will be, my soulmate, my best friend and my hero. I am so grateful to him for never once failing to help me realize what truly matters. There is nothing I am more grateful for in life than having him by my side.

I also want to express enormous thanks to my own mentor and coach, Jayne Morris, who helped me through the worst times and continues to be my mentor. She helped me to climb out of that hole and back into the light and, in truth, changed my life.

# Foreword

For decades, the most widely available health and fitness information geared toward women has been produced primarily by the multi-billion dollar weight-loss industry—an industry that preys on our insecurities for profit. This industry is unrelenting in its efforts to convince us that we aren't good enough, thin enough, lean enough, or pretty enough, and wastes no time rushing in to sell us "solutions" for all of our shortcomings.

It's no wonder so many of us feel like we're forever a "work in progress" or like we're just not "there" yet (wherever "there" is, for any of us). From a very young age, we are blasted with messages that tell us that in order to be worthy of love, success, happiness… worthy of living a life we love, and even worthy of loving ourselves… we first have to achieve a certain physical ideal. We punish ourselves, we tear each other down, and we keep ourselves stuck in place, waiting for the day when we have earned the right to live out loud, the right to be happy with ourselves, and the right to feel good in our bodies.

These messages are so ingrained in our psyche that we don't even realize it doesn't have to be this way until something—or someone—shakes us out of it!

Luckily, there are women like Heather Wynn, who are on a mission to transform the conversation for and about women and fitness. It's thrilling to know women who are standing up and fighting back against all the nonsense we face every day. Heather's compassionate and practical approach focuses first and foremost on the understanding that you can't hate your body into true health.

Heather provides simple and actionable steps to first help you shift your thinking, then your behaviors, and then how you feel, resulting in improved self-care practices that come from a place of love and reverence for your body and yourself. Through these practices, you'll gain sane and sustainable health and physique changes, from the inside out, and finally arrive at a place of peace and love, of which you've been worthy all along.

Heather's entertaining writing style and insightful anecdotes from her personal journey as well as her professional work with clients, help us recognize the absurdity of the expectations for our bodies that we allow outside influences to determine for us, and the type of lifestyle we think we need to live in order to be healthy and fit.

After reading this book (actually, maybe even just ten pages in!) you will feel empowered to step off the diet roller coaster for good, quiet the negative voices, and reclaim your life and health. The best part? Heather will give you the tools to do it!

Molly Galbraith

Molly Galbraith is the owner and co-founder of Girls Gone Strong, a global resource for women's health, wellness, nutrition, training, and lifestyle information, uniting hundreds of thousands of women from over 60 countries across the globe. Girls Gone Strong is changing the way information about health and fitness is presented to women, providing evidence-based, body-positive information, using a united voice to silence the fear-mongering, multi-billion dollar weight-loss industry and mainstream media who prey on women's insecurities for profit.

# Part One

# 1

# Introduction

One summer evening, I found myself on the phone with my good friend Angela. She filled me in on her recent birthday night out.

"So I ordered the chicken. I wasn't sure what it had on it, so I scraped the sauce off and ate it plain. I did eat a spoonful of rice but then felt so awful because I was worrying if I'd had too many carbs. And rice is bad, isn't it? I managed to avoid the spring roll we had for the starter because of the pastry, as I wasn't too sure what it had been cooked in. It might have been vegetable oil and that's *really* bad, isn't it? I only drank water because alcohol is awful and has carbs and sugar, but everyone else drank the champagne. They all said they'd all had a brilliant night, but to be honest, I didn't really enjoy it that much. But at least I was good. I wasn't naughty; I was good. Wasn't I?"

I've heard people talk a lot about their so-called 'epiphanies.' I wasn't sure if I'd ever had one up until that night, but this conversation signified the first of many to follow. I put the phone down and reflected for a moment. How on earth had it come to this? When had it become the norm that this level of restriction, fear and guilt around food had become a viable way to live?

Although I'd had similar thoughts regarding clients in the past, this was the one that provoked me into taking action. It was probably due to the fact that I was impartial, as Angela was speaking to me as a friend and I had stepped out of my professional bubble. As I started to recall similar conversations with my clients, I realized that these scenarios were no longer as sporadic as they had once been. The type of language that Angela had used about her food choices was becoming much more widespread.

I was appalled. Not only because it became clear that my friend thought that I'd be pleased that she had gone out and had a thoroughly rubbish time, but mainly because she'd been encouraged to behave this way by her current coach.

Okay, so he may not have said the words "Go out and have a thoroughly rubbish time," but the list of rules, guidelines and checklists that he had etched into her mind as being the only 'healthy way to eat' had subsequently impaired her thinking. His teachings had rendered Angela's own instincts and common sense redundant.

Originally, she'd approached her coach for some help in order to feel a little healthier, give her a bit more energy and lose the few extra pounds that had accumulated on a recent holiday. However, within the space of just a few months on the plan that the coach had recommended, she had gone from being a confident woman who was able to cook, eat and take care of herself—with the odd overindulgence every now and then—to what I can only describe as (sorry, Angela) a dithering wreck around food. She'd become completely obsessed about what she was and wasn't allowed to eat and her coach had managed to convince her that she needed to behave this way around food if she wanted to stay healthy.

Straight away I understood what was going on inside her head. I could clearly see that she was on a very slippery slope. She had started off as someone who shared a healthy curiosity for nutrition but was rapidly changing into someone who had an unhealthy and unnecessary fear of food. I knew this to be the case because there had been a point in my life where I had felt this way too. Even as a coach, I had previously been sucked deeply into the new hip and trendy 'clean eating' movement. At one time, I too had started to slide down that same slope towards obsession, leading me to the point where I would spend the whole day feeling anxious if I knew I was going out to eat somewhere new.

If you're reading this book, chances are that you will at some point in your life have felt that if you could just lose some weight, then everything would be better. You may have felt that if you could just be slimmer and look like the women on billboards, then you would finally be able to do all those things you've always wanted to do but never did because you felt too self-conscious. You might have in your mind this picture of a shining thinner version of 'you' whose life is just so much happier than yours, a smaller you who feels cool and confident and can cope with life so much better.

This hope and expectation of what weight loss can give to you can quickly escalate into a cycle of addiction, fear and anxiety. Perhaps you started off on a short-term diet plan 10, 20 or even 50 years ago, and now here you are still searching for that next diet plan promising to bring you all of those things. You're addicted to the quick fixes, the new fad diets, the celebrity-endorsed exercise gadgets, and potentially, subconsciously, you may also be addicted to the coaches who promise you that these things will work.

Having worked within the diet and fitness industry for over 16 years, I've learnt so much about the way the industry works and about the people who buy into it. The truth is, unfortunately, the industry isn't always out to help you. In fact, often, it really doesn't care how you feel; it cares about how much you spend. And what's the best way to get you to spend more? To make you feel worse about yourself, of course, so that it can sell you a new way to make you feel better again!

This statement may make you feel confused and even feel protective about the industry, because the consensus out there is that funky fad plans and exercise gadgets are all about helping people feel healthier, lose weight and become better people. To be told that this isn't always the case may evoke defensive feelings within you because it's been something you have trusted in and believed in for so long.

Way back in my early twenties, when I was on my first-ever personal training qualification course, my tutor said to me, "You are not selling them the diet and you are not selling them an exercise session; you are selling them a *dream*." Each time you buy into a new diet fad, a coach who promises the earth in 12 weeks or a new extreme exercise trend, you're buying into that dream. The dream being sold is never specified beforehand, because it's personal to you. The dream only exists in your head because it's made from the emotional connection that you bring to the table. The dream is made up from that *one thing* that you think weight loss will bring to your life, that one thing which you haven't got now.

The diet industry draws you in because it promises to fulfill that dream, our innate desire for self-love, confidence and contentment. You keep buying into new diets simply because the media keeps you convinced that a new diet has what you need to experience these things. Subliminally, the diet industry whispers to you that weight loss holds the key to true fulfillment in your life.

Behind the scenes of this dream-selling business, the widespread use of fitspiration and shaming disguised as motivation continues to break down any confidence you have, crushing whatever self-esteem you had so that it can promise to build you back up again by changing how you look. With enhanced images and deceptive advertising tactics, you are convinced that if you work hard enough to look like this vision of 'ideal' then you too could be happy, confident and feel amazing every day.

Sadly, when it comes to the diet and fitness industry, it seems that we have lost all of our common sense and logical thought processes. If it was so good at what it did and if it actually delivered on the promises that it promotes every day, then the results achieved would last a lifetime and it would effectively eventually bankrupt itself. The truth is, the multibillion-dollar industry thrives on repeat trade.

If there was one real, effective, single-track method towards sustainable long-term weight loss, their so-called promises would be fulfilled and their market share would diminish and eventually crumble.

When you get stuck in the mindset that your weight is the be-all and end-all of your worthiness, you make your whole life about that one-dimensional view of yourself. Whatever plan you may have in your head about what you want to do in life, your weight is made an integral part of that plan. You might be using your weight to bargain with—"I'll go for that new job when I've lost a kilo…"—or other things you want to do that you justify not doing on the basis that you need to lose weight first. You may seek out similar reasons as to why this belief is true, adding to your own confirmation bias that if you can just "lose this weight" then your entire life will change for the better as a result. I have sat in front of clients who've refused to take a holiday for five years because they haven't lost specific amounts of weight in order to do so. They look upon this physical change as the Holy Grail that will lead them to fulfillment, freedom and ultimate happiness.

Losing weight for the sake of health alone is rare these days. There is nearly always an emotional link to what you feel weight loss will bring to your life as a result. On the surface, you may *believe* that you want to lose weight to simply become healthier. However, subconsciously, chances are that you will also be buying into the dream that a smaller dress size will have the side effect of making you happier with who you are.

You aren't to blame for wanting to believe that this dream is real. That's why I've written this book, after all: to help you understand how you got to the point of believing that all your worth depends on the number inside your jeans. It will become clear to you just how you've become so caught up and obsessed with the ever-expanding world of diets and weight loss, and how you've got to the point of feeling so resentful about how you look, so guilty about everything you do and so fearful of what you eat that you don't really know who you are anymore.

At some point in your life, you have been sold the dream. Just like thousands of other women out there. Just like I was.

Through the course of this book, I'll take you behind the scenes of the diet industry with a backstage pass! It'll become clear just how you went from being a confident, smiling and self-assured woman to someone so afraid of her own body that intimacy has since become more akin to the *How-To Guide for Keeping Your Pajama Bottoms on While Having Sex*.

I'll explain to you how the once-simple task of getting fitter and feeling healthier can more often these days leave you feeling the complete opposite of what you signed up for and, more importantly, I'll help you to protect yourself from falling into this trap ever again.

The obsession with weight loss that has led you to the obsession with dieting is not because you have 10 pounds to lose; it's because the industry has convinced you that losing 10 pounds will make you happier. It's also likely managed to convince you that, whoever you are, whatever you do, you are not and never will be enough as you are.

My job over the course of this book is to help you to escape from this limiting and life-controlling mindset, to move your life forward in a positive, confident and empowered way. Over the course of Part One, I will be offering you information designed to open your eyes up to the truth behind the smoke and mirrors of the health and fitness industry. There may be parts that you are shocked by, but I only feel this to be a positive thing. I am going all-out, no holds barred, because I want you to know the whole truth.

I understand that you need more than just information and behind-the-scenes gossip. You also need practical help in order to make this journey count. So, in the second and third parts of this book, we will delve into what it really takes to create long-lasting change within you and how you can achieve real confidence and experience that elusive self-love that you crave without having to put yourself through the trauma of trying to fit in with the gym crowd while pretending that you really love eating kale for breakfast. I will show you how you can start, straight away, to put the wheels in motion towards the life that you want rather than the life that you *think* you ought to want.

By the time you've turned over the last page of this book, you'll have finally begun to understand that what you are really searching for cannot, and will not, be found in a smaller pair of jeans. Self-love, acceptance and worthiness are already there, waiting to be found within yourself, whether you wear your 'good day' jeans or your 'bad day' jeans.

The power behind everything that is currently holding you down, keeping you hostage as a fully paid-up member of the yo-yo diet club, will be made redundant. You will be able to move forward with your life, safe in the knowledge that never again will you have to buy into that expensive box of magic pills, quick fixes, or gurus in order to feel at peace with who you are.

Before we move on, with a view to helping you get into the mood for what is to come, I would like to share another epiphany moment with you. It was another phone call; this time, however, it was with a client, a woman who I'd just started working with. She was what many people would describe as inspiring because she was tall, toned and had a naturally slim figure, indeed matching up to that ideal that is supported and promoted in our contemporary culture.

On this day, Miss Inspiring was in floods of tears down the phone to me. Having refused to go out that day, she'd informed me that she just wanted to go to bed to "get away from it all." The trigger to this enormous meltdown? Well, she was unable to see her abdominal muscles in the mirror. She had let her family go out without her and, instead, was on the phone crying to me about how terrible this made her feel. The worrying part was that, as time went on, it became obvious that this episode was not a one-off for her. This lack of ab definition was something she worried about on a daily basis. This level of obsession unfortunately isn't unusual, but the overriding point I need to make here is that she had the type of figure that many of my other clients would have listed as their goal 'I want to look like' physique because, in their eyes, having this kind of figure would provide them with undoubted and unwavering confidence. What they don't see is that this desire to be 'more' truly is a never-ending cycle of misery.

There is an element of humor in stories such as these and, yes, you would be forgiven for thinking they are coming from prima donnas who have nothing else in their lives to worry about or from women with pre-existing disorders. Still, I want you to understand that this just isn't the case. The majority of clients that I have worked with who have felt like this have been intelligent, hardworking, sane women with families and responsibilities. The unhealthy relationship with food, the destructive body obsession and the emotional turmoil that I have witnessed in so many women—all of which stems from the incessant pressure to conform to the 'ideal'—isn't reserved for the wealthy and bored among us. Absolutely not. This is a very real scenario for millions of women worldwide.

I feel strongly that it's time things changed, and I know that change is possible...and right now, right here, that change starts with you.

## 2

# Why I Wrote This Book

As I progressed through my career within the health and fitness industry, it became very evident to me that the majority of the women I came across were living with a chronic and debilitating lack of self-esteem. I spent so much of my time listening to the derogatory language that women use when describing themselves that I really have heard it all. Most women openly speak worse about themselves than they would ever about their worst enemies. Having to watch so many amazing women hide in the shadow of their own lives, because they felt completely unworthy of anything that the world had to offer to them, was just heartbreaking.

Many I spoke to would turn down opportunities and walk away from joyful experiences or activities because they had convinced themselves that they were not good enough to take part, or because they so fiercely feared the criticism and judgment that might come as a result of showing up and 'being seen.' I'd speak to women who'd spent years justifying the decision not to follow their dreams on the basis that this life of self-limitation was them being realistic, when, really, it was all just another way of hiding from the fear of judgment. In their eyes, making an excuse as to why it's not possible for them to achieve something will save them from the perceived danger that they've attached to giving it a go and being criticized.

I came to the swift conclusion, professionally and personally, that most women in fact feel guilty about pretty much everything they do. It seems to have become a standard day-to-day emotion for many of us: guilt for what we do, guilt for what we don't do, guilt for how we do it, guilt for when we do it and guilt for who we do or don't do it with. The more and more I delved, the clearer it became that the majority of my female clients were spending their whole lives living in a way in which they *felt* they should live, rather than the way they wanted to live.

There was an undeniable air of unhappiness around a majority of my weight-loss clients, even those who didn't really have (in terms of health) any real need to lose weight. The common denominator with the majority of these women was that they fixated obsessively about how they looked. They all highlighted their physical appearance as something that they could perhaps change without a lot of effort (or so they thought), and this change seemed to them to be the quickest route to finding the master key to happiness they so longed for. As a result, the desire for physical change became the light at the end of the tunnel for them. There was a hope inside them, a voice that convinced them that if they could just get a better body, then all the other areas of their lives would become better too. They were adamant that their life would become exciting, they'd feel content and they'd finally get to experience that elusive feeling of being 'enough.'

But the sad realization was that, even for those who did achieve the physical change of weight loss, life didn't automatically become exciting again. Life was the same as it was before. They put all their conceivable effort into changing their physical shape, yet were still left searching for that sense of worthiness at the end of it. I witnessed this cycle over and over again. Even with a better body (in their eyes), apart from having to shop for smaller clothes, their lives would ultimately stay the same as before. They would still be waking up each day to go to the job they thought they *should* be doing, buying the things they thought they *should* be buying, impressing the people they thought they *should* be impressing, and living the life they thought they *should* be living.

After ten years of seeing this pattern repeating itself on a regular basis, it finally dawned on me and became a part of one of my many epiphany moments: these women weren't unhappy because they needed to lose weight; they were trying to lose weight because they weren't *happy*!

The once-imagined joy of living in a slightly smaller transport model (body) would quickly wear off once the before-and-after photos were posted and the compliments and validation from others had begun to die down. At this point, that initial buzz would diminish, the novelty would wear off and they'd reappear a few weeks later claiming that they just needed to lose a little bit more. Despite having convinced themselves for months that "if I could just get to 69 kilos" (about 150 pounds) they'd be forever happy and never want for anything else, here they were at 69 telling me that it wasn't enough. The goalposts had shifted to 65, then 63, then the desire to see more muscle definition, and a bit more off after that. It never stopped because each time they'd get to the end of the rainbow, they'd realize that there is no pot of gold waiting for them there; there is no fast-track ticket to internal peace.

However, true to form, clients would try to convince me that they were an exception to the rule. We'd have candid conversations about why they wanted to lose "just a bit more" weight and many promised that if I could just help them to lose this last bit *then* they'd be happy. In all my time within the industry, there have been very few clients who would reach a weight-loss goal and simply enjoy the feeling of being there without the immediate need to create a new, more extreme target.

This was summarized perfectly by a lady who contacted me recently. She was right in the middle of this scenario when she contacted me in response to a blog I wrote. I'll let her share with you her story in her words:

"When I began this process, I felt that if I could lose weight I'd become this confident, happy-go-lucky person. But all the self-judgment I'd had previously just shifted onto other areas. I'd watch other women in the gym and think *No matter how much I try, I'll never look like that.* I don't feel massively different from how I did before. There will always be that voice there telling me I'm still not good enough."

The nutrition and fitness industry should be entirely focused on adding to people's lives in a positive way, physically, emotionally and mentally. However, it has become apparent to me over the years that, unfortunately, it has started to play a key role in actually diminishing our self-esteem and sense of well-being. As I spent all those years listening to the scathing ways in which women would view themselves, I could see clearly where it was stemming from, and it was partly down to the advertising and media that surrounded my industry—the one that was supposed to be helping. So it has now become my passion to help people like you, like me, and like my clients, to free yourself from the constraints of an industry that falsely convinces you that your worth as a woman is determined by your dress size.

# 3

# The Facts and Stats

Let's start by looking at a few facts that will help me to explain to you why it is that I believe the health and fitness industries is failing women.

The diet industry is a $59.7 billion dollar industry and it's getting bigger and bigger every year. Many predict that this figure will reach $100 billion by 2017.

A recent WHO report stated that 74% of men and 64% of women in the UK will be overweight by 2030.

It is estimated that obesity costs the UK National Health Service (NHS) over £1 billion a year, and if you look at the cost to the country as a whole (through such things as work absenteeism and benefit payments), then this rises to £3.5 billion a year. If you consider this and then factor in all the co-morbidities that go with obesity (such as diabetes, heart disease and hypertension), it is expected that obesity will eventually bankrupt the NHS.

On the other side of the pitch:

A quick search via Amazon will provide you with access to over 100,000 diet books, and that number will surely continue to grow.

On any given day in the USA, 25% of men and 45% of women are actively on a diet. In the UK, the average 45-year-old has been on 61 diets, a survey has found. The Boston Medical Center indicates that approximately 45 million Americans diet each year and spend $33 billion on weight-loss products in the pursuit of a trimmer, fitter body.

We now have more qualified personal trainers, fitness professionals and nutrition coaches than ever before. It has never been easier to become qualified as a fitness or nutrition coach or to set yourself up as a well-being expert. We have more research being done and access to more information than we ever had.

So it's strange that, when you start to compare our health statistics with these facts, it is clear that as a society, we are bigger, less healthy and unhappier than we have ever been. These statistics shouldn't make any sense though, right? We have more people and more resources than ever trying to fix the problem, yet the problem just keeps getting worse. How can this possibly be the case? If the industry were doing its job, the statistics would be showing the evidence by now.

# 4

# Missing the Wood for the Trees

What you currently believe to be the root cause behind these health statistics will all depend on what camp you have received most of your dietary education from. If you have favored the Paleo diet for example, then you'll have most likely been convinced that sugar or grains are to blame for these shocking statistics. If you've been on the Weight Watchers journey, then it will be dietary fat that is at the route of the problem. Vegans will tend to blame meat. If you have preferred the Atkins approach, then the blame will be placed firmly at the door of all carbohydrates (I feel that this has merged into Paleo in recent times). You may feel it's just plain laziness and a lack of movement that is to blame, a deficiency of willpower, or possibly even the fault of the giant supermarkets which place sweets and other tempting offers in our eyeline at the checkouts.

Everyone has an opinion as to just what is at the root of this failure to gain control of our health and well-being.

The truth is, we can't just pin down any one reason, but that doesn't make for a sexy and outrageous headline. So the media choose to grab onto anything that they can create a sellable story around, usually something that will appeal to our apparent need for something to blame.

As a result, in my experience, most people will all too happily cling onto each latest diet fad that has been rolled out, as they are cleverly convinced that this new approach will finally be the thing to fix their problems. Even after having adopted numerous different approaches in the past, all with the same expectation, people still tend to believe that this newest diet will be the one that cures them forever.

As a coach, I have worked with clients following each and

every one of the different diet methodologies. Some fared well from certain diets and others, not so well. There is no 'one size fits all' scenario; just because it works for one person does not mean that it is guaranteed to succeed for the next. If there was one diet out there that could make us all slim, happy and healthy, then, trust me, we'd know about it by know.

In fact, *JAMA: The Journal of the American Medical Association* has actually advised us to stop researching diets:

> The long history of trials showing very modest differences suggests that additional trials comparing diets varying in macronutrient content most likely will not produce findings that would significantly advance the science of obesity.
>
> Progress in obesity management will require greater understanding of the biological, behavioral, and environmental factors associated with adherence to lifestyle changes including both diet and physical activity.
> JAMA. 2013;310(7):687–8

All of the different diets have their place, to a certain extent, but I think we need to get honest about this now and start to lay it down for people that there is no one diet for all. The best diet out there is simply the one that leaves you feeling good—mentally, physically and emotionally—and that you can adhere to for the rest of your life. Apart from that, there really are no set-in-stone guidelines.

Being honest, I don't believe that the problem is down to a lack of education, as many coaches like to cite. I think given the chance, most of you reading this would be able to write out an example of a pretty decent diet plan if I asked you to. Most people have a pretty good idea as to what constitutes a healthy-*ish* diet and what doesn't. I saw a recent survey which asked two very simple questions about weight loss and dieting. The options were:

A. I don't know how to maintain and keep my body healthy. [or]

B. I know what to do but just can't seem to do it.

The unanimous responses were for B, and I can imagine that you may agree with that also.

However, this is where I believe it becomes more difficult to discern what the answers actually indicate. I wonder just how many women who answered that question with B actually already had a healthy body, but were mistaking health for the wish to be slimmer? We have to be honest with ourselves at this point and admit that, in truth, most women don't embark on each new diet with the hope of simply improving their health. This yo-yo diet cycle you have gotten stuck on hasn't been born from your desire to live until you are 90; it's been born from a desire to change the way you look.

It seems that the health and fitness industry have forgotten what health really means. Health these days has become all about being good-looking.

# 5

# But I Need to Be Slimmer to Be Happy!

Throughout this book, I am going to be completely upfront and honest with you. There will be parts that I could have left out for fear of being criticized and could have judged myself for including. But this book is dedicated to helping you and the best way that I can do that is to be totally candid about the journey that it took to bring me here. The first thing I'll admit is, going back a few years, I understand that I may have unintentionally let clients believe that the meal plan I was giving to them or the exercise program I had put together for them was going to make them slimmer and therefore better people. But I wasn't alone; the health and fitness industry continues to give away this impression to its clients every single day.

I knew that these people were coming to a coach to find the answers to their body problems that they were assuming would lead them to happiness and acceptance. As I look back at some of the information forms that I used to ask clients to complete before coming up with a plan for them, the majority of answers I received about short-term goals tended to be along the following lines: "to lose weight," "get smaller," "be slimmer," "have visible abs." However, next to long-term goals, it would often simply state "to be happy."

This was evidence that so many people had bought into the dream that weight loss will bring happiness. When a client comes to a coach for a diet plan, it's often evident that this search for happiness is at the core of their decision to reach out for help. The trouble is that there is no real correlation between happiness and weight loss. This is not just my opinion and it is not just anecdotal: it has also been identified in studies. One such study done by University College London (UCL) states: "Weight loss over four years in initially healthy overweight/obese older adults was associated with reduction in cardio-metabolic risk but no psychological benefit, even when changes in health and life stresses were accounted for."

Another study was done more recently that found similar results. The lead author, Sarah Jackson of University College London, wrote:

> We thought that if we excluded healthy-weight individuals from our sample, which previous studies showing adverse consequences of weight loss had failed to do, we would see positive changes in mood with weight loss that mirrored findings from the clinical-trial literature. However, this was not the case; even when we restricted our sample to individuals who were overweight or obese, and would therefore be recommended to lose weight, participants who lost at least 5 percent of their body weight were significantly worse off psychologically at our follow-up assessment than those who maintained their weight.

One of my personal theories, based upon my personal experiences, is that this connection could be a result of taking away what was once a major source of enjoyment and fulfillment. Many people look upon food as a release, an emotional safety net, in the same way that some people do with alcohol, smoking, etc. They know they are guaranteed to get some type of joy from it; they take pleasure from it no matter what else is happening in their lives. It could be the only source of pleasure that a person has in their daily grind. In fact, I have seen this to be the case many times.

Another highly likely reason is that the increased feelings of depression and reduced well-being are born from the vast disappointment that dieters are exposed to as they fail to find the expected happiness as a result of weight loss.

I can absolutely back up these findings. As an example, one of my previous clients came to me with the aim of losing a bit of weight to look slimmer (as she wants to remain anonymous, we'll call her 'Sarah'). She wasn't substantially overweight, and, in fact, according to her doctor, she was healthy in every way with every box ticked. However, Sarah felt that she ought to look a little slimmer.

Her day-to-day routine consisted of working very long shifts with lots of overtime. She was single and had no children, so therefore felt working was making good use of her time to keep active and pay off her student debts. However, at the end of these long shifts in a job that she didn't particularly enjoy or get any fulfillment from, often she'd come home and reach for a glass or two of wine and a chocolate bar to enjoy while relaxing. It was her downtime; she enjoyed this part of her day immensely and it was clear from her doctor's report that it was having no adverse effect on her health.

During the course of our initial session, it became apparent that the really obvious way that Sarah could go about losing the specified amount of weight that she felt would make her happy with herself would be to cut out this habit of chocolate and wine. She would have to change her food choices or take up a new hobby to relax with—one that didn't involve food. This would be the route that the majority of coaches would tend to adopt, emphasizing the willpower-based approach.

However, when we discussed the potential for change regarding these habits (i.e. changing her routine or even just her food choices), her jaw dropped. She was horrified. This daily indulgence was her salvation and she looked forward to it immensely. However, she did not refuse to make the changes.

When I considered Sarah's situation realistically, it dawned on me that if I demanded she went down this obvious route, then I would be telling her to effectively cut out the only source of joy that she currently felt in her day. Just cutting out this pleasurable part of her life, without working on the root cause—which was her overall day-to-day feelings of fulfillment—was never going to be the long-term solution. To see change in someone's life to the point where food is no longer used as the only source of pleasure takes time and effort and cannot be done via a well-scripted nutrition plan and a few motivational emails.

This isn't an unusual case; women all over the world are out there actively trying to restrict joyful experiences in their lives in order to buy into this view that 'smaller means happier.' It's ironic that, in the hope of feeling better, often the very food or experience that they cut out in order to do so is one of the true sources of pleasure they have in their lives. At that level, of course it's going to fail. It isn't a diet issue; it's a lifestyle issue. The root of the problem lies in the fact that, apart from food, there is very little other joy or fulfillment in their day-to-day lives. If we stop obsessively trying to take away that last source of enjoyment in order to see quick physical results and, instead, actively work on increasing the experience of fulfillment elsewhere, then eventually the need for that food as emotional gratification will diminish over the long term.

I want to put a disclaimer in here and stress that I am in no way saying that I feel it's a bad thing to want to change your diet *or* body shape. I am a coach through and through, so of course, I will always advocate health at every level. If you know your body will function better at a lower weight or you've been advised by your doctor to lose weight for health reasons, then by all means pursue what will ensure a healthy future for you.

What I do want you to understand, though, is that achieving that lower weight will not automatically make you happier. In fact, the actions needed to achieve that weight loss may even make you feel worse. It may make you healthier—if done the right way with balance and flexibility, no fads, no unnecessary food restrictions and taken up from a logical place within you rather than an emotional one—but it will *not* automatically lead you to the catalogue-image 'I'm running down a beach in a bikini and everything is awesome' life that so many expect to gain from it.

So, talking about this bikini-beach-awesomeness, let's dig into this expectation a bit further. We'll assume that it's you who likely thinks that you are the exception to the rule, as you believe that losing weight will be the answer to your dreams. I guess you've probably embarked upon diet after diet and yo-yo'd your way through many, losing a little here and gaining some more there. Each time, the willpower fades and the rules become too much and you end up slipping back where you started. But the feelings that started it all are still there, so after a while, this kicks off the search for yet another magic pill or secret trick, something that you are convinced you may have missed along the way. My first question to you here would be this, in brutal honesty: *Why didn't it last?* There would have been at least one time in your life that you lost weight, maybe one time that you got to (or near to) your goal weight. So why didn't you maintain it? Did it not make you happy being there? Think about this for a second. If it did make you happy, surely you would have done anything you could to stay there?

Losing weight is like a failed relationship. We think back and recall all the good bits, conveniently forgetting about all the arguments, the bad days, the irritations and all the effort that it took to make it work. When your relationship starts to come off the rails, you try to rekindle it on the basis that all you can think about are the good times and you tell yourself that you are sure that you were exaggerating the tough times. It's only when you get to the same point again that you remember why it didn't work out last time. It's exactly the same with yo-yo dieting. Each time you have lost weight, you didn't find that pot of gold at the end of the rainbow. You didn't find it because it didn't exist. If you had found it, you would have been very committed to holding onto it. Therefore once you *were* there, you felt you needed to go further to find it—the goalposts of happiness had moved. Each time the goalposts move, the diet becomes that little bit more restricted and unsustainable. Hence, the inevitable fall off the wagon that leads you to head right back to where you started.

Please understand that I have to talk like this. It is absolutely not a dig at anyone who has recognized this pattern. Whether you think it's harsh or blunt, at this point I want you to be aware that I am more concerned about getting to the truth than I am about protecting your feelings. That's not to say I don't care. I do immensely. It's like what your parents used to say: I'm doing this because I *do* care. I'm doing this to try to help you understand why it is that 95% of your diets have failed. It's because 95% of *all* diets fail, so no matter how many more you go on, they'll likely fail too.

When we talk about diets failing, it either means that weight loss is not achieved at all or weight is lost but then later regained. So let's be honest, if weight loss gave to people what they'd initially hoped for, then we'd be looking at a *success* rate of 95% for diets. If we had found the gilt-edged route to peace, confidence and happiness via a diet, then you would think that the majority of dieters would do anything they could to sustain that feeling once they had found it. But they don't. The diet happens and nothing changes, apart from fitting into a smaller pair of jeans. The novelty of having to restrict and control food intake to sustain that smaller pair of jeans seems to be tremendously hard work when compared with the rewards that they'd originally hoped for.

# 6

# So What Really Leads to Happiness?

The crux of the matter is this: the life that you live, day to day, has got to make you happy. Happiness is a state, not a destination. If you are spending your days on a diet and exercise regimen that makes you feel like you want to suffocate yourself with a yoga mat, then, first of all, you have to admit that you aren't enjoying the journey. And if you aren't enjoying the journey, then it's time to recognize that you aren't likely to enjoy the destination either. Most people on diets tend to forget about the endgame. All too often it's conveniently forgotten that the task of maintaining a loss when you finally reach it can be just as hard as the journey it took to get there. As a quick-fix hunter, you are likely convinced that once you shed all your desired weight, you'll just automatically be able to maintain it with little to no effort. This tends to be where it all goes wrong, because the initial weight loss is the easiest part of the long-term journey (note how I said *easiest*, not easy!).

Once it starts to sink in that a dream packaged in a sparkly new diet plan isn't all it's cracked up to be, then it will become much easier for you to open the door to other ways in which you can make positive changes to your life. Previously, you may have ended up becoming completely blind to the other things that are affecting your confidence levels, because you've spent so much of your time blaming your weight for everything. But, once that blame has gone, opportunities will present themselves which will enable you to identify far more effective routes towards achieving that true, authentic confidence and self-love.

## 7

# I Should Be So Lucky

Have you ever met anyone in your life who never, ever, had weight issues? You know the ones I mean: those who whip out a doughnut in the middle of a meeting without a second thought and go back for double helpings on apple pie day, without that whole "Should I? Shouldn't I?" conversation, with seemingly no physical repercussions. I'm talking about those people whom you envy for their ability to be able to eat anything they want but never seem to gain weight. Apart from the physiological reasons (higher basal metabolic rate (BMR), higher energy expenditure, lower intake overall, etc.), these people are also more likely to have a logical relationship with food, whereas by now I think you'll have started to recognize that you're likely to have an emotional one.

When these people grew up, they likely did so in a house where food or weight was never really discussed in an emotional sense. You may think that this would make them more likely to gain weight if they were in an environment where they were not forced to diet or restrict their food intake, but this is precisely why they don't have the associated problems stemming from an emotional need for food. Food is logical to them; they think about it with strategic, clear-cut and reason-based thought processes, eating being just something that they 'do' without overthinking it. This is because, as their subconscious mind developed, food wasn't used as a replacement for love, neither was it given or restricted as a result of good or bad behavior. They were taught to see food as fuel; of course, they still enjoy eating and have tastes, but the emotional response to food is just not the same. Furthermore, body weight (thus a secondary effect of food consumption/restriction) was never used as a judgment tool of self-worth.

So, what happens in the opposite scenario: growing up in a house where food and weight is talked about constantly and emotionally? Perhaps becoming used to having sweet treats when you'd been good, leaving a subconscious feeling that this type of food provides you with the comfort of being loved and nurtured for good behavior. Perhaps if you were feeling down, your parents or grandparents may have given you a cake or sweets to make you feel better, again leaving you with an association that cake and sweets made you feel better, that they act as a comfort. Maybe you were also used to being praised when you lost weight and ignored when you gained weight, so your natural quest for love and connection became a game attached to what the scales said. Perhaps you were denied your favorite food when you had been naughty or given your favorite food to keep you quiet? All of these situations can mean you now associate specific emotions with what you eat. This subconscious emotional connection can be the whole reason behind your need to reach for the chocolate or the wine or the crisps (or all three!) when you've had a bad day; it can be the voice behind the justification when you say "I deserve it!" as you tuck in to an extra slice of pizza; it can be the driver of the difference between you eating until satisfied and eating until you feel sick.

Why, oh why, do we expect ourselves to be able to simply turn off this subconscious connection as soon as we become an adult? The media, the diet industry and maybe even your coach seem to expect that you can just click this part of your brain onto 'mute.' As you are growing up, your subconscious mind spends its time sucking all this information in like a sponge. Unfortunately, you cannot pick and choose what it absorbs and you cannot switch these messages on and off as and when you want. As a result of these teachings when you were younger, your subconscious mind hangs onto this information and drives your behaviors, actions and decisions in response to it. This part of your brain will continually remind you that a cake or sweets will make you feel better when you are down and it will tell you that you deserve an extra slice of cake after receiving good news. It absolutely doesn't respond to the logical words of your coach who sat there telling you to just "stop doing it." Unfortunately, your subconscious mind is infinitely more powerful than your coach.

The good news is that there is absolutely no need for you to completely cut out chocolate and wine after a bad day. Heck, we all enjoy this kind of treat to a certain degree. The key to just how destructive these habits become is based on whether or not you can honestly answer these questions with a firm 'NO' response:

- Do you find it hard to control yourself when you eat these foods?
- Does your emotional response to food have an impact on your health?
- Do you often feel the need to have the whole bar *and* the whole bottle in order to get the benefit of that emotional response?

If you can't answer 'no' to all three, that is when the behavior begins to turn from being harmless and part of a balanced and flexible lifestyle to becoming potentially destructive and controlling. Once again this is not going to be fixed by a diet plan.

If you answered 'yes' to any of these questions, it becomes important to understand what emotional response this food is providing you with. Is eating the only time you experience a sense of true joy and happiness? Does eating give you the only sense of fulfillment you get in your life? Does it stop you from feeling lonely? If it does, then, like Sarah, you are bound to end up eating more than you really need to, because it becomes about filling an emotional hole rather than a physical one, which can be never-ending. In situations like these, even the best and most expensive fitness and nutrition coaches out there will be unable to create a plan that will stop you from doing it. If they do, then they will effectively be removing that last ounce of joy and fulfillment that you have control over, which may work short-term, but is it any wonder that these plans fail eventually? It's a form of torture, not motivation.

The subconscious beliefs that are the root of this emotional relationship to food in the first place are where the focus needs to lie in order to achieve long-term and sustainable change.

It's not just your family who have their hand in creating your subconscious beliefs around food and dieting. These subconscious connections are continually reinforced every day by the diet and fitness industry itself. The industry plays on this idea that it's all to do with finding the willpower to just stop overeating. It gets its claws into you and makes you feel even worse by convincing you that you are just lazy and that it's your fault that you can't stop eating more than you need. It is also your subconscious that is in charge of your belief that in order to be worthy of love and acceptance you need to be, look or act a certain way.

I know, you're probably in a state of flux right now as I've just told you not only that happiness can't be found in a smaller body, but it can't be found at the bottom of a biscuit barrel either. So, you may ask, yanking on your hair, where *is* it to be found? Well, without sounding all cliché and soppy, it's to be found within yourself. You can't 'get it' elsewhere, unfortunately. These external places of satisfaction that I have spoken about (whether it's eating cake to feel better or fitting into smaller jeans to feel better) are merely fleeting. It's just the same as expecting that new car or bigger house to do the same thing. A true feeling of authentic happiness will be found through contentment in your day-to-day life, living in accordance with your values, appreciating your talents and character, forming authentic personal connections and contributing to the world. Your self-worth, which acts as a precursor to this happy state of mind, needs to come from within you. It's there already; it just needs to be found, built and appreciated. The later sections of this book are dedicated to helping you to do exactly that.

# 8

# Your First Diet Fix

Let's take a minute to go back in time to where it all began: that first diet fix that got you to fall hook, line and sinker into the physique-focused world of yo-yo dieting.

Most of the people who I have worked with have followed a similar path in respect to their first diet fix. Let's see if yours follows it too.

Usually the story starts with you paying a bit more awareness to how you look. Perhaps something got your attention in the media or you saw an advert in a magazine that made you glance down at your thighs and deem them 'not acceptable,' becoming concerned about them being too big or the wrong shape. Once this feeling has been activated, you perhaps start talking with other people about how you feel, who may also admit to feeling the same way as you do. One of these people, at some stage, will no doubt begin to pipe up about an "amazing" new diet or "fantastic" new supplement that they have discovered and that they are planning to try. This sparks a decision within you to try it too.

On the other hand, it may well be a professional who sparks your interest. For example, if you are already a member of a gym, it may be the coaches or other trainees around you who introduce you to this 'new way to lose weight.' Either way, a conversation will result in you coming away with some type of new diet idea, tablet, drink or exercise trick. No sooner than you have left the conversation, it will become etched into your mind. You have been sold the idea that this is 'the one,' and you simply have to try it. The media and clever marketing around you can also be heavily involved in drawing you into that diet cycle as well. Over time, they continuously subliminally encourage you to question yourself and the way you look, making you a prime candidate for this new, fantastic weight-loss method. Essentially, you are being primed your whole life, so that when this inevitable conversation happens, it takes less than a few minutes for you to end up agreeing to give it a go.

Once you are committed to embarking on this new 'diet *du jour*,' of course you throw yourself into it. On the outside you convince yourself that you are onto a winner, as you tell your friends and family (and yourself) that you are feeling better than ever. But on the inside, a different story is playing out. The pressure you are under to see it work makes you stressed, obsessed and anxious, and your self-esteem begins to deteriorate to the extent that you may even feel worse about yourself now than when you first started this stupid diet. Rather than your logical brain taking over and reminding you that this should be making you feel better and, in fact, you never felt this bad about yourself before, your emotional brain runs the show by telling you that the reason you are crying more is just because you are just not thin yet.

However, the truth behind these tears, anxiety and despair has nothing to do with the way you look. You looked the same before you ever even started to diet, and felt okay. It's because your self-esteem is slowly being crushed by the pressure to conform, the pressure that you bought into that very day you started the new diet.

It's so easy to get sucked into this cycle and, unfortunately, the longer you stay in it, the harder it is to escape from.

It doesn't help that some parts of the industry seem to think that you feeling bad is conducive to greater success. Sadly, many coaches have seemed to adopt the attitude that berating, yelling and judging someone has become an acceptable way to motivate them. So how are you meant to know that feeling worse about yourself isn't right? How are you meant to be able to pull yourself out of this self-perpetuating hole if the coaches around you are the ones pulling you back in? Sadly, actually—*appallingly* seems a more appropriate word, these days—there is a distinct possibility that you will walk out of a gym session with far more self-hate than self-love. In gyms all over the world there are people being shamed and criticized into pushing themselves harder and in more extreme ways, constantly being made to feel that they aren't good enough while being treated like schoolchildren when they don't follow the specified 'rules.'

If a client has a genuine need for weight loss, it's essential to evaluate that person as an individual and it's up to the coach to decipher what the key driver is behind the desire to eat that is creating the need for a diet in the first place. It has been shown time and time again that shaming isn't an effective motivational tool; in fact, more often than not, it has the opposite effect. Alternatively, if the client is *not* overweight, but still insistent that they want to become slimmer, then the focus should be on identifying the real reason behind this need for physical change to ensure it is coming from a healthy and emotionally secure mindset.

Unfortunately, many coaches very rarely take any of this into account or even register it as important. Instead, you are likely just scooped up at the door, given a list of rules and regulations detailing the 'good' and 'bad' foods, how much you are allowed to have and at what time, and in less than an hour you have been thrown head first into the 'show-me-your-dedication' tornado— no ifs, buts or maybes about it.

Despite clutching all the rules, regulations, lists and set routines that your legs can carry, your subconscious eating behaviors and the subconscious drivers behind your perceived 'need' to lose weight will always still be there, just waiting in the wings to trip you up. The fall from the wagon is inevitable and, should you be unfortunate enough to be around the coaches who shame in order to motivate, then you'll most likely be cast aside and labeled as 'too much trouble' quicker than you can utter the words "I just had a bad day…"

If we all—coaches, clients and everyone else on the planet—were to be just a little more focused on building up our and others' self-esteem, then the falls off the wagons, the yo-yo cycles and the need for the quick fixes would begin to dissipate. If we, as individuals, spent more time looking for meaningful fulfillment and less for external validation, we'd no longer be totally consumed with judging our self-worth on how skinny we were. Also, we would no longer need biscuits or crisps or wine to fill the emotional void. Find true fulfillment and, suddenly, life opens up to you and you no longer care whether or not you can see your abs that day (if ever). You'll begin to experience things that will give you a deeper sense of satisfaction, while recognizing that you were only obsessed with your abs and/or food because there was nothing else in your life you wanted to focus on.

It's time to let go of this conditional self-love that you've anchored in yourself. Your self-worth isn't based upon how you look; it is based on how you *feel* about the way you look. It is time that you began to recognize that how you feel, right now, is entirely within your control.

The sooner you drop the conditional love for yourself and realize that you are worthy of love and acceptance as you are, the sooner the diet and fitness industry loses you as a repeat customer and the yo-yo stops yo-yoing.

# It Starts with WHY

Most clients enter into the dieting process with complete and utter faith in the industry. They place full trust in the coaches and the methods advised to them. They place all their hopes and dreams into the hands of the coaches, who promise to provide them with all the tools they'll need to change their body. But of course, having now recognized that thoughts, beliefs and the subconscious rule behavior, not 'willpower,' it's only a matter of time before many inevitably start to falter and begin to slip back into their old habits. Far, far too often, clients are then blamed for "not wanting it badly enough" and are criticized in the gym circles for "not having what it takes." This falter and slip phase is more commonly known as 'falling off the wagon,' as mentioned earlier, and it happens mainly because the behaviors behind their habits and self-limiting beliefs have been left to fester without being addressed, but it can also happen if the plan they are attempting to follow is outrageously restricted and unsustainable. When the advice given is all rules, restriction and 'cut-out' approaches, there are bound to be persistent falls off the wagon; a falter and slip for any of these reasons suggests that the client absolutely isn't at 'fault' in any way. If anyone, it's more likely the coach is at fault for still believing that willpower is all it should take.

I have witnessed clients being shouted at for not sticking to the plan by their coach, and being spoken to like a three-year-old who is about to be placed onto the 'naughty step.' It's mortifying to witness, and horrifyingly, the motive behind many of these chastising sessions is often to do with how they were making the coach look stupid by not getting results. The client, in the meantime, has already been banished to the bargain bucket of self-worth and will, most likely as a result, just retreat back into their shell with increased feelings of failure and even lower self-esteem than they had when they first started.

One of the issues in the industry that I've noticed has grown over the years is that the industry is so saturated with coaches all so desperate to attain guru-status that they prioritize their business and reputation over the individual clients. If a client looks to be one who won't make a good before-and-after shot for their wall, some will actually refuse to work with them. Not only is this hugely irresponsible and unacceptable for an industry that is supposed to be about health, but once again what it is doing is re-emphasizing that the only thing that matters in life is how you look. You can't tell a person's health, mental or emotional state from a before-and-after photo, hence the reason I stopped doing these years ago. This isn't a generalization, as the majority of coaches do not act like this; however, I do know that it does go on, and if you ever end up on the receiving end of any coach's narcissism, I implore you to have the confidence to just walk away.

Anyone who consistently struggles with their eating habits should be encouraged to look deeper in order to understand the thoughts and beliefs behind the behaviors that keep them locked in this yo-yo cycle. The focus should not be on how one diet is better, but rather why there is the need (and whether the need is physical or psychological) to diet in the first place.

An example highlighting this point well was seen recently in a social media group that I am a member of. It was written by a lady who could be described as a typical yo-yo dieter. By this, I mean that she had spent a large proportion of her life on diets, never really seeing any consistent success, thus constantly searching for the next one. She said:

Okay folks, help required please and will be gratefully received. Can anyone show me a typical meal plan for a day? Need some advice on how to structure my meals. I eat 3 times a day, always eat breakfast and am pledging to STOP SNACKING when I'm not hungry. I'm changing my workout routines from pure cardio to a mix of body pump, shred and meta fit. My resting heart rate is 54, and I'm aiming to lose around 10 pounds then maintain. Thanks loads!

From the quote, it is clearly evident that she knows part of the problem is that she eats even when she is not hungry. A problem that many clients have when they approach a coach for help— they eat in accordance with what their mind says as opposed to what their stomach says. However, here you can see she is still convinced that she needs a new diet plan in order to fix the issue, showing a great example of how common it is to believe that a new meal plan will be all that is required to make behaviors better.

This belief is in no way unusual! These sorts of questions are posted in social media groups or pages every day. The reason behind these requests, and the reason behind the success of 'cookie-cutter' coaches (those who sell non-individual meal plans), is the fact that the majority of yo-yo dieters crave this sort of instruction. They want to be told exactly what, when and how much to eat. This is why the large slimming clubs have such great member retention, as they provide their members with a step-by-step instruction manual and tell them exactly what they can or can't eat, but they don't deal with the behavioral or psychological side of things, creating prime candidates for repeat trade.

In order to succeed at this thing called health, yo-yo dieters are convinced that they need a detailed guide of how and what to eat. Keeping ourselves healthy is one of the most basic and fundamental tasks we have as human beings. It should be something that we do instinctively. However, because we have spent years and years being told that whatever we are doing, we are doing it all wrong, we now have diet clubs and coaches queuing up to hand out new instruction manuals about how we should eat. As a result, this has created a huge amount of paralysis by analysis; many people no longer trust themselves to be able to eat well and stay healthy without the aid of a coach.

# 10

# Ready for Change

Time for honesty again. I used to give clients everything they asked for, including the menus and instruction manuals. A list with example meals all planned out and calorie-counted. Carefully thought-out exercise plans with periodization, progressions and adaptations to keep them interested. When I was writing meal and exercise plans, I'd catch myself justifying foods or exercises to the client, already worrying about them pulling a face because they saw the foods as boring. I was convinced that it was my job as a coach to make this world of optimal nutrition more interesting for them. I wanted to make their food plans more exciting and make their exercise programs as stimulating and varied as possible to help them stick to it.

Another one of my epiphany moments came just as I was writing out yet another list of suggested meals for a client who hadn't even remotely stuck to the last three diet plans I'd prepared. As I was sitting there, it suddenly dawned on me that my role was becoming much more akin to that of a primary school teacher. I was having to coax and cajole clients into following the advice and instructions that I provided—the instructions that, to begin with, they so desperately demanded and had convinced themselves they needed. Writing the plan had become the easy part; the hard bit came when I had to convince the client to actually follow it. I needed to devise ways that would ensure that clients could put the written plan into action.

Coaching in this industry can be truly exhausting; it really can. To be honest, I am going to qualify that statement—it should read 'coaching *well* can be exhausting.' As a coach, you are so much more than simply a diet advisor or exercise plan designer.

You become your client's friend when an argument with a partner makes them eat an extra biscuit. You become a counselor when they want to know how, next time, they can stop themselves from eating that extra biscuit. You become their parent when you are having to bribe them into following the plan for a full week, promising treats of extra puddings or wine if a plan is adhered to. You become a teacher as you have to justify why you are asking them to increase their activity levels or spend a full hour dissecting why it's not sensible to fast all day in order to have an alcohol binge at night.

You constantly have to encourage, motivate and direct, not only to keep things on track in a practical way, but more so in an emotional sense. I feel it is extremely difficult to be able to coach well without getting involved in a client's life beyond what they eat, because so often over/undereating is a symptom of something else going on under the surface that no amount of willpower can fix. The need to be constantly coaxed and cajoled into making changes often happens because, quite simply, you just aren't ready for change or because you are just trying to focus on the practical 'eat less' admonishment rather than the root cause of why you overeat in the first place.

I dealt with many clients who'd turned up to the coaching process before they were really ready for it. Many times I turned people away and instead referred them to therapists, psychologists or specialists. Many times I should have done so but didn't. Again, very rarely is their state of readiness even looked at before the client is sent off with a new diet plan and shopping list. It's important to understand that not everyone is at a state of readiness for change, and also, not everyone really wants what they *think* they want.

Dr Gary Mendoza, PhD, specializes in assessing stages of readiness within weight loss clients. The following offers his important insights into the whole concept of readiness and lifestyle changes:

**Are you ready to lose weight?**

There are many diet programmes that all claim to be the final answer when it comes to weight loss. They all claim to be easy to do and that you can eat what you like and the weight will fall off. The truth of the matter is that they are all doomed to failure. Even if these promises were possible (they're not, by the way) they are all missing a key element, namely that of behaviour change. My mantra when working with clients is "it's your lifestyle that got you fat and only changing your lifestyle will get the fat off (permanently)".

Lifestyle change is not easy, you are trying to undo years of conditioning. My research highlighted that quite often people enter a weight loss programme but they are actually not in the correct stage of change psychologically. Because of this it is inevitable that the programme will ultimately fail and the weight will return. The transtheoretical model for change was first hypothesised by Prochaska and DiClemente in 1983. This model incorporates a number of behaviour change theories, including the stages of change model, self-efficacy theory, decisional balance, and the processes of change. The stages of change model hypothesises that when you make a behaviour change you go through a number of stages on your way to successfully making a permanent change.

The stages of change include pre-contemplation, this is where you are not thinking about making a change and in this stage you are unlikely to enter a weight loss programme. That said, people in this stage of change can enter a programme due to peer pressure or perhaps for social/family reasons. Because they are in pre-contemplation they psychologically don't want to enter the programme therefore they will ultimately drop out. The next stage is contemplation, in this stage they are weighing up the pros and cons of losing weight. What they ultimately feel at this stage is that there are most probably as many pros as there are cons. Again from a psychological standpoint they are still not ready to lose weight. Next comes preparation, by now the pros may outweigh the cons and generally this person will enter a weight management programme within a month or so. From here they move into action and start the weight loss programme. Approximately six months after entering the action stage they may move into the final stage, maintenance. This very much depends on how much weight they needed to lose.

The importance of this model is that my research has highlighted that if you are not in the correct stage of change then ultimately any weight loss attempt will fail. The other factor is that even if you are in the right stage of change initially you can still relapse at any point. When a relapse occurs you can move back to any of the previous stages (including pre-contemplation). This is clearly demonstrated by serial dieters who have tried numerous FAD diets. One thing you have to take account of with these individuals is that it is quite possible they were starting each new diet cycle in the wrong stage of change. Therefore they were doomed to fail from the outset. By assessing an individual's readiness to change you can greatly enhance their chances of success. What is more this monitoring should continue throughout the programme to ensure that psychologically they are staying in the correct stage of change.

A very simple assessment you can do is write down all the pros and cons for losing weight before you start your journey. Start with a blank A4 sheet and try and list as many cons as you can for losing weight. There are no rules here so if you think it's a negative then list it. Often this list will include things like, I'll always be hungry, I'll have to give up my chocolate, you get the idea. So give free rein to your thoughts and be brutally honest, list everything. Now give yourself a break for an hour or so and get a fresh A4 sheet. Cover up your cons sheet, in fact file it for the minute. Now list all the pros for weight loss, again give free rein to your thoughts. When you have finally exhausted this thought process compare your pros and cons, providing the pros greatly outweigh the cons then you may just be ready to change. This process is fairly basic and there are psychometric tests available that will measure all elements of the transtheoretical model for change. I have utilised these tests as part of my research and when training personal trainers. I have found them to be an effective tool for assessing whether people should enter a weight loss programme. If you are psychologically ready to change then your chances of success will be significantly higher.

—Dr Gary Mendoza, PhD, Mentor, The Nutrition Academy; Lecturer, Bath University

# 11

# My Early Coaching Years

Allow me to take you back in time to where it all began for me personally, as a person and a woman, as well as a coach, so that you can understand how I got to be writing this for you today.

Throughout my teens and early twenties, I wasn't comfortable with who I was. I spent my teen years feeling physically and emotionally insignificant. Ever since primary school, I'd had this underlying feeling of unimportance. I used to think that I resembled a 'Moomin'—a cartoon character—because of its facelessness. Whenever I was out in public, I felt featureless and believed that if you moved more than a few feet away from me then I would just blend into a big round blur of nothing. If I was out and someone from the past recognized my face, I would genuinely feel surprised. In fact, I was so convinced that I was utterly and completely forgettable that I would sometimes hide from people so that I didn't have to endure the whole toe-curling scenario of the other person asking, "Sorry, what was your name again?"

So, in my early teens, I figured out that if I pushed myself more in the gym, thought more carefully about the food I was eating and embarked on the path of body perfection, then I was bound to become recognizable and memorable. I would become someone to remember.

At the age of 17, I began my career in coaching and threw myself into the job of helping others, which I hugely enjoyed. I was good at coaching so that was what I focused on. It became a massive part of my life almost immediately. However, when I wasn't with my clients, my thoughts would always return swiftly back to myself again and each day. My thoughts and fears, my obsession with perfection—these were becoming stronger. I now had an image as a coach to keep up with; I wanted to be seen to walk the talk. And no matter what I did, I was always wanting, needing, to be better. Up until recently, I can't remember ever being truly comfortable with who I was. Of course, many of my clients felt the same way too, as did many of my colleagues. So, because I was with like-minded people day in, day out, it quickly became the norm to live in this world of self-deprecating thoughts and conversations, leading to extremity and restriction that was disguised as dedication.

As I look back, it was strange that when I was working with clients, I would always become aware of the danger signs when they were taking things too far. If I had a woman who I felt was getting a little too obsessed, I'd tend to be on it straight away and I'd manage it well. For clients, I used the mantra "You can be a little obsessed, but just not *too* obsessed"; for myself, though, there were no such boundaries in place.

However, it's clear to me now that, compared to many people I have seen and worked with since then, I wasn't actually as obsessed as many of the clients I see today. I have absolutely no doubt that this obsession with body-fixing and dieting has gotten far, far worse over the last ten years.

Clients would look up to me and they'd constantly assume things about my health. "You must feel amazing with all the exercise you do and with how healthily you eat…" At the time, of course, I'd reply with beaming smiles and lots of flamboyant hand movements to confirm just how absolutely amazing I felt. But, in truth, I didn't always feel so good. I had no respect for the fact that my mental health had just as much of an impact on how I felt day to day as my food and training plan, so subsequently, I ignored that side of things. I was entirely focused on the physical aspect, as I believed that it was the be-all and end-all of everything. I had bought into the dream myself, the dream that I was then selling on to others.

# 12

# Fads, Promises and Secrets

Open any magazine, walk through any gym and scroll through any social media platform and you will see just how bombarded we get with diet-related jargon and buzzwords:

- six-week-abs
- secrets
- tips
- nutrition rules
- fat loss foods
- quick fixes
- power foods
- detoxes
- gut health
- gimmicks
- gurus
- body wraps
- fat burning
- juices
- smoothies
- calories
- eat clean
- gluten-free
- high-intensity interval training (HIIT)
- cardio
- grain-free
- vegan
- raw food

You will have no doubt been exposed to at least two or three from this list over recent years. If you've ever been on a diet, you'll most likely have been given a list of things to cut out of your current diet or been provided with a list of rules to adhere to regarding your eating behaviors. None of these nutrition plans, methods, ideas or promises will ever be guaranteed to work for you—what could be one man's meat may be the next man's poison. There are also no slimming or fattening foods. One slice of 'fattening' cake will have absolutely no negative effect in the context of an otherwise balanced diet. A 'slimming' food is just as likely to result in fat storage as a 'fattening' one if the food is eaten in excess.

This is why I am going to spend some time helping you to decipher the warning signs to look for when embarking on any new health kick (notice I said *health* kick, not body-fixing-diet-kick). I know that there is a chance that you may still get tempted to go down this route in the future, as I mentioned earlier. This approach isn't designed to put you off from looking after your health as a priority; it is designed to help you *separate* your feelings of self-worth from how you look or what you eat (or don't eat), and instead view your health habits in a practical, logical and long-term sense, with no attached conditions pertaining to your overall feelings of self-esteem.

This will near enough eliminate the need for any quick fixes or guru-magic promises or secret potions, so it's important to recognize whether you are looking at a genuine long-term, sustainable idea to help improve your health or a gimmicky, 'selling you the dream' type, appearance-centered method disguised as health advice.

If a coach tells you within your first meeting that you have to eliminate an entire food group from your diet, and you haven't got a genuine medical reason for doing so, then I'd implore you to think twice before taking their advice as gospel. Of course, your own common sense prevails here—if you have to sprint to the bathroom every time you eat a sprout, then no need to eat sprouts, yay!—but cutting out a specific food-group is often completely unnecessary for health *or* weight loss and is also a behavior that, in my opinion and the opinion of many fellow coaches, can be the trigger that encourages disordered eating and possibly even nutrient deficiencies.

Almost every woman I have helped with disordered eating behaviors stemming from food fears and anxieties (including myself) began the journey by first labeling foods as 'good' and 'bad,' then moved on to start eliminating specific food-groups entirely. The only people that genuinely need to eliminate entire groups of food for long periods of time are those with certain religious beliefs and those with diagnosed medical conditions, sensitivities or allergies. Always refer to your GP (family doctor) or a registered dietician if you are concerned that you are reacting to a certain food. If you truly are experiencing intolerance symptoms from certain foods in an adverse way, then this needs looking at as a priority since simply cutting out foods will not solve the problem long-term.

In Part Three, I will talk more about getting to grips with critical thinking to help ensure that you don't get caught up in these fads and gimmicks in the future.

For now, just take a moment to look back over your dieting history. How many different protocols have you been sold? Most women I have asked this question have been able to immediately come up with at least four, but I would suspect that the real number is higher. You have been sucked in to these trendy ideas because you have always been completely convinced that there is still something somewhere that you are missing. Your belief in this hidden secret is what the diet companies, supplement reps and advertising platforms use to get your attention. A new diet catches your eye and you are drawn into it immediately because it contains some type of 'hook.' By a hook, I mean it gives you the impression that it's a new idea and it contains the hint of something you haven't tried before, making you think that this is why you have never succeeded in the past, because you missed this one detail that this new diet has to offer.

You buy into it, you start it, and all seems well for a few months as you feel relief that you've finally found the plan, the one that has all the answers and is everything that you have been searching for. Chances are that you'll possibly lose a few kilos, maybe even more. However, soon enough things start to become a little tougher. The food begins to feel a bit mundane, you feel yourself getting a bit bored and the novelty starts to wear off a bit. You get tired of eating to a set of rules and find it harder and harder to stick to it. That little voice in your head starts to pipe up, chirping away in your mind that "There must be an easier way." The plan goes out the window, most likely without even a hint of a logical decision being made. It just drops off and fades away. You look around a month later and wonder what the hell happened, but you shrug your shoulders and justify it with "Life is too short to diet anyway," and proceed to start making up for the last few months of rabbit food by eating with total abandon and no concern for what you eat or why you eat it.

But six weeks later, your jeans are feeling a little tighter, you have no energy and that all-too-familiar feeling comes back. You start thinking to yourself "Why didn't I just carry on?!" Before you know it, *ta-da*, you are sitting in front of your computer again tapping 'lose weight quickly' into Google, rebooting the cycle all over again.

I don't want you to feel bad, in any way, if some of what I have just described resonates with you. Truly, I would imagine most people reading this can recognize that scenario in some way, shape or form. But having the ability to recognize these yo-yo cycles in your own past behavior is the first step in releasing yourself from it happening again and signifies the first small step toward the start of a new, empowered journey.

## 13

# When Healthy Becomes Unhealthy

I discuss disordered eating a lot because I feel this subject needs to be opened up more, especially for those who either are most at risk of suffering from disordered eating habits or are around those who do suffer from them. Those most at risk are those already involved in weight-reducing behavior and appearance-fixing habits (dieters). Coaches themselves can be at risk personally, since they are likely to witness these behaviors in and around their places of work.

There is still a large stigma attached to disordered eating and it makes it hard to discuss openly without fear of offending or upsetting. Still, it's a very real problem that affects many people and, with the advent of a new and potentially misunderstood eating disorder, sometimes people are suffering without them even recognizing it.

Orthorexia is a relatively new addition to the eating disorder family, introduced officially in 1997 by Steven Bratman, MD, MPH. He describes it as "a medical condition in which the sufferer systematically avoids specific foods that they believe to be harmful."

Wikipedia describes it as follows:

*Orthorexia nervosa* (also known as *orthorexia*) is an eating disorder characterized by an extreme or excessive preoccupation with avoiding foods perceived to be unhealthy. The term 'orthorexia' derives from the Greek ορθο- (ortho, "right" or "correct"), and όρεξις (orexis, "appetite"), literally meaning 'correct appetite', but in practice meaning 'correct diet'.

Before I go on, I feel it's important at this point to mention that general healthy eating isn't to be confused with orthorexic behaviour. Steve Bratman clears up the often-blurred line between disordered eating and simply wanting to eat well for health:

> Enthusiasm for healthy eating doesn't become 'orthorexia' until a tipping point is reached and enthusiasm transforms into obsession. Orthorexia is an emotionally disturbed, self-punishing relationship with food that involves a progressively shrinking universe of foods deemed acceptable. A gradual constriction of many other dimensions of life occurs so that thinking about healthy food can become the central theme of almost every moment of the day, the sword and shield against every kind of anxiety, and the primary source of self-esteem, value and meaning. This may result in social isolation, psychological disturbance and even, possibly, physical harm. To put it another way, the search for healthy eating has become unhealthy.

During my own brief stint of orthorexia in my late twenties, my obsession focused on sugar, toxins, sweeteners and pretty much everything considered not clean. As my obsession around food started to build, so did my already problematic anxiety. I had suffered with anxiety issues since I was a child, at which time I was going through therapy for GAD (generalized anxiety disorder). As I started down the path of this new 'clean eating' trend, I was not only convinced that it would make me lean, happy and free from disease, I was also convinced that somehow my anxiety would also be cured. I had been taught (by well put together, cherry-picked evidence-based sources) that sugar was the absolute root of all evil and that anything that entered my system that hadn't just been plucked from the farmer's field itself was immediately going to harm me—oh, but then there was the pesticides and the GMOs, so it needed to be an organic farmer's field. I was convinced that if I ate 100% natural and whole foods, all of my worries and anxieties would disappear and I would be as healthy as a person could be. Well, that didn't happen and, in fact, things got worse. At the height of this obsession, my anxiety went through the roof, most likely due to the fact that I'd added so many other things to my list of stuff to be fearful about, as well as because I was avoiding so many foods that it became just impossible to live a normal life.

I was suckered into this world myself even after having already been a coach for ten years, so I can easily see how the general public falls into the fear-of-foods rabbit hole so easily. There are scaremongers everywhere just waiting to inform you that what you are eating has been linked to a multitude of diseases. If you look hard enough, you can find an article, blog or theory about pretty much any food on the planet being bad for you! We even have gluten-free water selling now, because apparently nothing is safe. There will always be someone sitting in the next seat on the bus or your mate who read the paper that morning who wants to tell you that what you are eating or how you are exercising is all wrong and that there is a better way. Until the new *new* better way comes along next week, that is.

Talking about diet and health at social occasions became another source of anxiety for me. Which was weird, considering that previously I had loved talking to people about what I did. I was always passionate about my work and enjoyed the conversations that it brought up, but during this blinkered time my passion became rigid and narrow-minded. The more obsessed I became, the more I became closed off to any opinions outside of my own. It would immediately rile me when people asked about why I was eating a certain way. I'd get defensive and feel as though I was being personally attacked. Of course, I wasn't. People are curious and due to the fact that most people knew I was a coach, I'd always be asked questions. It was only natural. Even so, I'd always try to steer the conversation away from the subject of nutrition, which is partly still true to this day, but not because it makes me anxious; rather because it is still never a good idea to debate food with friends or family, as it's impossible for anyone to be completely correct—and many just can't comprehend this level of uncertainty in something so complex. It becomes akin to a religious 'meaning of life' type of debate…and we all know how heated those can get!

I'd climb on top of my high horse whenever there was even a glimpse of food in the vicinity, crinkling up my nose at how awful most of it was. Away on holiday, I'd view the breakfast buffet in hotels with absolute disdain because of the lack of protein or 'real food' choices, becoming like a petulant child, huffing and sighing as I skulked past the pastries. In fact, I'd often choose to go without eating, even if this meant that I would potentially not eat until the evening, if it meant I could avoid the 'toxic' foods on my avoid list. The psychological worry of eating a 'bad' food was far worse than the physical pain of hunger. Similarly, if I was to stay over at a friend's house, it was embarrassing to have to sit at a breakfast table where they had laid out a lovely spread of fresh breads, jams and croissants, and pretend that I wasn't ravenously hungry, that I was fine with just water.

It is quite right that no one should ever have to justify his or her food choices. We shouldn't and I'm not suggesting that you ever do. We are all free to eat how we like. Once again, people who have serious allergies, sensitivities and genuine dislikes of certain food should never have to defend what is on their plate or why they would rather not eat. My motto these days is "eyes on your own plate" and I feel that is the take we should all have. I would never suggest you need to eat something you don't want to just to please everyone else but, and there is a big but, I *do* feel that it becomes very important for you to be totally up-front and honest with *yourself* when justifying the way you eat. The responsibility lies with you to be able to look deeper inside and ask yourself the real reason why you refuse to eat a slice of bread. You have to be open, able and willing to recognize the warning signs of obsession or disordered behaviors, which can be hard when you are in the midst of it, as you'll likely defend your choices vehemently until something somewhere triggers a need for change.

I always justified my food decisions as being totally health-based during those years, but when I got really honest with myself, of course I knew deep down that having a slice or two of toast every few weeks was, quite honestly, not going to harm me. The whole health argument becomes a bit redundant when you realize that some of the healthiest nations on earth eat these foods you fear for breakfast every single day. Ironically, it's quite often the very nations who eat these foods that put all of the USA's and UK's health statistics to shame. The health justification was nothing but a cover-up for the fact that, psychologically, I was unable to deal with eating the type of foods that I'd perceived to be inherently 'bad.'

As I've already mentioned, no food is bad in its own right. Any food should always be viewed in context, however. Another sign that you are in the grips of orthorexia is that dosage and context becomes completely irrelevant.

If you have recognized any of this behavior in yourself, I'd encourage you at this stage to open yourself up to the possibility that this 'health' line you speak has potentially become your cover-up story for something that has become more psychologically driven than physical, just like it did for me and has for many others. Consider the following questions; the more you answer 'yes' to, the more likely you are dealing with some level of orthorexia.

- Do you wish that occasionally you could just eat and not worry about food quality?
- Do you ever wish you could spend less time on food and more time living and loving?

- Does it seem beyond your ability to eat a meal prepared with love by someone else—one single meal—and not try to control what is served?
- Are you constantly looking for ways foods are unhealthy for you?
- Do love, joy, play and creativity take a back seat to following the perfect diet?
- Do you feel guilt or self-loathing when you stray from your diet?
- Do you feel in control when you stick to the 'correct' diet?
- Have you put yourself on a nutritional pedestal and wondered how others can possibly eat the foods they eat?

Orthorexia is not only a condition that is affecting more and more of the clients and customers of the health and fitness industry, it is also highly prevalent among coaches who are placed in charge of looking after you. Many instructors in fact use this 'clean eating' movement as an acceptable way to hide their disordered eating habits. It makes it possible to pick, restrict and label food as good and bad. Most worryingly, this behavior is often seen as normal within fitness circles, making it extremely easy to cover up. However, the dangerous result of this is that we now have young influential girls being coached into 'bikini-ready' shape by someone who is suffering from disordered eating habits herself. I know of a number of coaches stuck in the ravaging cycle of an untreated eating disorder, who are right now advising other young girls about what they should and shouldn't eat. As time goes on, more and more are opening up with their own struggles.

Diana Kidd, an Australian personal trainer, has herself escaped from the grasp of the disordered eating habits that resulted from 'clean eating' pressures. Here is a snippet from her story that she shared when asked a very common question by a client:

Q: I want to lose weight. How do I cut sugar from my diet?

A: I started my weight-loss journey by cutting sugar...That turned into cutting dairy and fruit...That turned into cutting high-sugar veggies and grains...That turned into only eating organic...That turned into only eating local organic...That turned into growing my own vegetables, only eating eggs from my hens, only buying particular meat from a particular butcher...That turned into only having ten or so foods I deemed 'safe'...

I had a 'birthday steak' instead of birthday cake...I took Tupperware containers of my 'safe' foods everywhere with me...I skipped social events with food...I didn't eat at family Christmas gatherings...I never ate at restaurants...holidays were a nightmare...

There are way worse things than having a little sugar in your diet—the resulting disordered eating behaviours and orthorexia from believing it is necessary to eliminate foods in order to lose weight can cripple your life.

The only time a food or part of a food is unhealthy is if we eat too much of it (excess) or, like in the case of carbohydrates currently, too little (lack).

Both excess and lack contribute to nutrient deficiency and can contribute to macronutrient and caloric imbalances—and that includes eating too much of a particular 'good' food, which then hinders variety in your diet.

So, the answer is, balance and health are what you seek, and through that, you will achieve weight loss. The mental side of weight loss is as important as physical fat loss and health. You need all three.

The ideal way to lose weight is to learn to understand the way in which all foods can help you achieve your weight and health goals, while avoiding a poor relationship with food and disordered eating behaviours.

Eliminating and restricting foods leads to fear, guilt,

shame, binging, suffering and perceived moral superiority — none of which will help you achieve your goals, and all of which will hinder long-term weight maintenance.

Fear-mongering is the enemy, not sugar.

If you feel that something, anything, in this section has resonated with you, please understand that there is help out there. I would always have to advise that your first conversation be with a trained eating-disorder therapist or psychologist, but I know from experience that most people showing signs of orthorexia will not feel comfortable in admitting they may need therapy. If this is the case, then there is not a whole heap we can do about this until you are ready to admit that this healthy living idea has gone too far. Like anything, you have to first be open to the possibility that there is a problem and you have to be ready to openly admit that it's starting to make you feel worse about yourself, rather than better. If you aren't there yet, then you won't benefit from being forced down the recovery or therapy route. But at any stage, if you start to wonder if you have crossed that line then please, *please*, don't try to sort this out yourself.

## 14

# The Penny Started to Drop

At the end of this period, I was tired, I was sick and I was also majorly confused. I couldn't understand how, after eating so well and being so active for so long, I didn't feel the way that I was supposed to feel. My genuine passion for health and fitness had resulted in me feeling like a wrung-out zombie and I knew that it was time I took the control back.

Over the next few months, I started to get better. I was allowing much more flexibility back into my food choices and, eventually, the orthorexic behaviors started to diminish. It was such an incredible relief to be able to eat the foods that I had shunned for so long. The first time I ate a piece of warm crusty bread, I can remember absolutely savoring every bite.

However, even though it was no longer associated with food, the underlying feeling of guilt and anxiety was still there. I now understand that, because I hadn't dealt with these feelings, they'd just moved around into a different area of my life. I simply transferred the control somewhere else and my work life was the next on the hit-list! This resulted in me overworking, never taking a break, feeling guilty for just about everything, and always going above and beyond, all to my own detriment. One step forward, two steps back! I was still stuck in the grips of an obsession, but now it just had a different focus; rather than food, it was 'hustling.' I still hate that word; it grates on me like fingernails down a blackboard. After years of this pattern, of one obsession just moving to another, eventually, I just completely burned out.

It was the breaking point and I ended up just throwing my hands up, letting go and making the call to take the time-out that I needed to in order to prioritize my own self-care for a while. This was the best decision I ever made. I sought proper help and this person spent four months with me helping me to unpick the beliefs and thoughts that lay at the root of all these obsessions and fears I'd been battling. Undeniably, a severe lack of self-esteem lay in the middle of it all. Low self-esteem is described by many psychologists as "the problem behind all problems," and this I absolutely believe to be true.

I spent months working on the stuff that had been clogging my mind up. It was truly amazing what came up—things that I'd never even thought I was bothered about ended up making me cry. I began to escape the clutches of everything that had been holding me captive in my mind, not just for the previous few years, but my whole life. The beliefs I'd had as a child about being unimportant, forgettable and 'Moomin-like,' all the fears and anxieties I'd just shoved under the surface—they had all played their part in my journey to that point.

I emerged with complete clarity and I was able to see my actions and behaviors in a totally different light. During this time, I'd also begun to recognize that the thoughts and beliefs that let me star as the lead in my own mini-meltdown were very, very similar to the thoughts and beliefs that I was seeing among my clients and other people around me.

When you are in the crux of it all and you truly believe you are doing the right thing for your health, you fully believe that everyone else has got it wrong. You think that it's truly acceptable to judge and criticize someone for drinking fruit juice or eating bread or generally eating any 'unclean' foods. A huge problem with this is that there is no real basis as to what even constitutes a 'clean' or 'dirty' food. It's totally subjective, therefore just laid wide open for contradictions and confusions. What is 'clean' to one person is totally different from what is 'clean' to another. This makes for disastrous consequences. So many people are watching these Instagram accounts from afar, reading the blogs and magazines, and listening to the guru-wellness-warriors, slowly but surely crossing foods off their 'allowed' list one by one.

## 15

# Where Is This Obsession Coming From?

Healthy became less about health and more about good-looking a long time ago. A new diet protocol advertised by a healthy but 5 kilos above 'media-ideal weight' woman would not get anywhere near the attention that a new diet advertised by a healthy but lean woman would get.

Now, this is where it gets interesting. I'm not quite at the level of advocating health at every size. There does come a point where body size does become detrimental to overall health and well-being, whether that be from obesity or emaciation. Luckily for us, though, this leaves a huge wide-open gray area to work with. You can lie anywhere on the scale in-between the two and be healthy. So this idea that the diet fads, trendy protocols and unnecessary restrictions are about health, I just don't buy.

The pressure to look a certain way is a key driver behind all these food obsessions. We at least owe it to ourselves to be honest about that, right? The thing was, as I continued on my path as a coach after my recovery, I began to realize that this pressure was no longer just coming from the catwalks, billboards and magazines; it had infiltrated from the core and was now bubbling up from deep within my own industry.

Skinny was out, strong was in, hurrah! But rather than sighing with relief, getting on with our lives and advocating every healthy body as an ideal body as it should do, the industry saw an opening. People wanted health, so no sooner than skinny was batted to the curb, healthy was brought in—except by this point, healthy had already started to morph into lean.

In every gym, leisure center and coaching studio, everywhere, a new pressure to conform had been born. The need to fit this new 'fit/lean/toned' ideal was becoming the new norm, all done in the guise of "but it's all about health now!" which really was just another way to make the old pressure to be thin a new, more acceptable advertising tactic.

Having already taken a step back from coaching, I just wanted to observe what was going on around me for a while and really understand just how it was all impacting so detrimentally on people's self-worth and confidence. I wanted to understand how and why so many intelligent women were being pulled into this world of obsession, fads and promises so readily and so easily.

I looked back over my previous clients, those who had succeeded in weight loss and those who hadn't. I revisited those who'd left me and gone off on their own and I spoke to many, many other coaches about all of this. Basically, I just talked to people and I listened, while switching off my 'logical' coaching brain. As a result came the epiphany moment that later resulted in my desire to share with others what I'd suddenly realized. The hunt to feel acceptance, love and worthiness was the number-one key driver behind all these diet obsessions, appearance-fixing behaviors and fear-based habits, yet dropping a dress size, seeing your abs or growing your glutes really has absolutely nothing to do with your ability to feel any of these feelings. As a result of this fruitless search, we are trapped on a hamster wheel going nowhere fast, too stubborn to get off.

I have witnessed clients lose more than half of their own body weight. I've been around many who have achieved extreme, life-changing physical transformations. I have seen people spend all of their spare income each month on weight-loss products, supplements or, more commonly, flitting between coaches trying to find the one who finally has the answers. The money that is spent on this search for weight loss is just vast. I've seen clients, friends and colleagues throw excessive amounts of money into the industry's pocket, as well as spending hours upon hours of their daily lives dedicated to this quest of leanness.

Around five years ago, I was a coach on a popular Sky 1 documentary series, fronted by Jessie Pavelka, a well-known US fitness celebrity. Over the course of twelve months, I helped an amazing woman shed 60 kilos; this loss equaled half of her starting body weight. The goal for the show was life-changing weight loss and she was one of eight contestants who all shared a similar journey. She succeeded. They all succeeded. Truth is, *many* succeed in this battle to see the needle on the scale move consistently to the left. Even so, if you look back a few years on, you'll find that the weight has returned for most of the contestants in the show. Now, this regain isn't a one-off, it's a recurring pattern happening everywhere. According to Gary Foster, PhD, clinical director of the Weight and Eating Disorders Program at the University of Pennsylvania, nearly 65% of dieters return to their pre-dieting weight within three years. As for those who achieve weight loss via a more restricted crash diet (diets that are severely calorie-restricted or include only a few foods), well, the statistics get worse, as only 5% of those on these kinds of crash diets will keep the weight off.

Whether you have a lot of weight to lose for health reasons or you are healthy but are convinced that you will love yourself more if you are slimmer, both situations show symptoms of low self-esteem. Something else is occurring psychologically. A journey that is started from a place of self-hate, self-destruction and inherent unworthiness is very likely to end with these feelings still intact. It has been shown time and time again that self-esteem is not born from how big or small your butt is; it's born from (among many other factors) your feelings of self-worth and how you perceive your value in the world. Basing this on how you believe you should look, and feeling as though your body shape makes you less worthy of love and acceptance, are symptoms of your own individual subconscious beliefs, ones that have most likely been growing within your subconscious mind since childhood. It is these beliefs that need the attention, as opposed to trying to fix the symptoms, i.e. fixing your appearance.

You could have the best diet plan in the world to help you to lose weight, you could achieve the leanest, slimmest, most attractive physical body you could imagine, but it will mean absolutely nothing in the long term if you do not have love and value yourself to begin with.

Self-esteem will not just improve on the basis of a physical change on the outside; it comes from the ability to appreciate yourself for who you are, unconditionally. It can be confusing and upsetting for some when the realization begins to dawn that self-esteem and its side-effect of happiness isn't something that we can buy with a credit card or just demand someone gives to us because we deserve it. We need to accept the fact that, scary though the thought may be, we are the only ones in control of how we feel and therefore how we live—no one but us.

# 16

# To Thine Own Self Be True

Going back to the point in my life when I'd just recovered from my burnout, of course I wanted to get back to work and I needed to, desperately—I was living on credit cards at this stage—and had to let nearly half of my client base go to allow myself the time to recover properly. Ironically and perhaps some may say crazily, this was also the point that my husband and I decided to pack up and move countries! The move was planned and we'd committed to our new home out in Spain, so we went ahead with it. I figured that it would be the perfect place to get myself together and figure out how I wanted to move forward with my coaching in light of everything. But I still had a decision to make. Honestly, I could have jumped straight back in to nutrition coaching and continued on that path, getting people lean or working them hard in the gym, writing 'food rules' and nutrition plans for people to follow and telling them how and why they needed to change— after all, I'd forged a successful career from this way of coaching and could easily have continued to make a good living from doing so. Or was I risking it all by staying true to myself and pledging to finish what I'd started?

This meant turning away from the looks-based coaching practices and the encouragement of body perfection; it meant putting myself out there in all my glory, standing up to the industry and yelling "STOP!" It was risky. I knew I was risking criticism and judgment and I had no idea if anyone would even be interested in what I had to say. But, hell, it was worth it. People started to respond, and the positive reaction was immediate. I began to put blogs, social media messages and short videos out there and I soon realized that I needn't have worried. There were many people out there who supported me and expressed their thanks to me over and over for highlighting the issues that they'd feared no one ever would.

I stopped prescribing meal plans. I stopped working with people who focused only on physical goals. I stopped talking about nutrition to clients who evidently had psychological issues surrounding food. I stopped talking about nutrition to clients who had body image issues. I eventually stopped taking on nutrition clients completely.

Instead, I began to talk to and work with clients in a different way, focusing on assisting people who wanted to get away from that obsessive lifestyle, those who wanted to improve their overall lifestyle, their confidence and self-esteem, without the prerequisite of weight loss. I started to help these women to find the strength to stop labeling foods as 'good' or 'bad.' I stopped demanding that people take part in exercises that they hated and, most importantly, I encouraged people to spend more time laughing and less time scrutinizing.

The amount of women who contacted me with their own stories of unworthiness, fear and guilt that had started as a result of an unsustainable diet plan they got wrapped up in with a goal of achieving this 'ideal' look was extraordinary. Not just ex-diet industry clients either, but coaches too. I began to focus the majority of my time on bringing these subjects to light, helping people in more meaningful ways. Now, here I am writing this book, wondering whether I could help the rest of the world to do the same.

My integrity is something that I hold close to my heart. It's one of my core values. I just knew that by staying quiet and cracking on as I was before, I would possibly even end up contributing to the demise of others, and there was just no way that was an option for me. There was never any doubt in my mind that the route I was going to take would be one of becoming part of the solution. As I stepped away from the old destructive aspects of coaching, I also released the part of me that had been gagged and held face-down on the gym floor, striving to conform to the expectation of a coach for the past ten years. I realized soon after that this part of me that I'd been trying to hide, the 'me' who refused to follow the crowd, was without doubt the *strongest* part of me.

My biggest regret in my time as a nutrition coach was unintentionally giving the impression that a diet, a weight-loss program or smaller clothes would automatically include a one-way ticket to worthiness and self-love. Even though I never specifically said it, every time I talked about dieting or fitness it may well have given the impression (even on a subconscious level) that weight loss would lead to happiness. The majority of coaches will agree with me that inner peace, self-love and happiness can never be found in a smaller dress size, but still, it's very easy for your words to say the opposite when you are involved in selling the dream.

# 17

# Gray Isn't Sexy

We all love black and white categories, don't we? We are always very keen to place every piece of information in either the black (wrong) or white (right) section in our brains. The public is bound to expect that the information provided to them by the diet and fitness industry is, without doubt, factual information that they can implant safely into the 'white' section of their brains. The seemingly logical thought process that many go off is that when health advice is written in the media, newspapers or is seen on the news, it is monitored and held accountable in some way. Most believe that because it's been written formally, the information must be right. Because of this, you believe that what you read in the tabloids or health blogging sites is all completely sound, backed-up and fact-based truth. These articles may even list a ruck of references with their theories, whether it's about the evils of a certain food, disease prevention or exercise advice. However, as the majority of us have not been taught how to decipher scientific research studies, then it's fair to assume that Jane Doe, who is reading the article in question, won't even click on to the listed references and read them, never mind under-stand them.

See, Joe Public relies on fitness and health professionals to decipher the scientific research and provide them with the relevant advice. Unfortunately, in the majority of cases, coaches are unable to correctly understand any of the studies that they come into contact with. The consequence of this is that when the information is relayed from coaches to clients, it takes the form of a Chinese whisper, the information being passed around becoming more and more exaggerated each time it is shared with another fitpro.

Richard Sennewald, a colleague and friend of mine, knows this only too well. He is a well-respected coach turned teacher-educator, whose ambition it is to effectively teach all his nutrition students how to correctly decipher scientific studies. Richard summarizes the situation perfectly as follows:

What I try to teach goes beyond evaluating a study. Learning, understanding and mastering critical thinking skills provides you with the tools to learn alone, without the reliance on a tutor (although a good tutor always has their place). The skills teach you how to gather data and to form your own opinions and how to challenge those to form your own valid conclusions, critical thinking and learning to appreciate the scientific methods that allow you to take part in intelligent discussion and present your ideas to others.

You see, the word of a qualified professional should be a solid and respectable thing, but in our industry, the nutritional industry, we lack a huge amount of quality control over who these 'qualified professionals' are. They could be a celebrity who stumbled upon weight loss, someone with an inspiring story where they overcame a health obstacle or someone with a little knowledge who is really good at writing.

Because we don't learn these skills at a younger age and seem to hold opinion with more respect than fact these days (because facts are cold, hard, emotionless beasts who care not for your rose-tinted views of the world), it is very easy to for example, read an abstract from a study or research paper, to read a blog from someone in the industry more practised than yourself who is a dab hand with the quill and to adopt their views as your own due to how convincing of an argument they put forward, which is all well and good...until that person is wrong.

To the person possessing no critical thinking skills, any argument is a convincing argument. This is the truth preyed upon by television spin doctors, media outlets and unscrupulous personal trainers vying to win you over through officious sounding statements, summary and conclusions that you, without knowledge of these skills, cannot interpret or dissect. This is partly why ridiculous diets exist, why celebrities are able to sell multi-million dollar book-guides to tepid lemon-water diets and why people who managed to run themselves sick and skinny can be online sensations carrying huge sway over the emotionally-charged diet industry.

Critical thinking skills are where experienced, researched fact and theory collide to create what is indisputably the best way forward for our industry. Without it, we are doomed to spend our days arguing about the latest pyramid scheme, quick fix and fad.

Richard's assessment brings me onto what I feel is one of the biggest problems within the industry. Essentially, how coaches are educated. Coaches tend to teach what the industry wants them to teach, but what has become clear to me is that what the industry wants us to teach is not always correct. I know that may sound shocking to you; the thought that coaches can and do teach things that are incorrect is quite frankly frightening. Even so, as an industry without any real regulation, coaches are pretty much free to do what they want. This issue becomes glaringly obvious when you consider just how many professionals within the health and fitness industry vehemently disagree with each other on some of the most basic facets of nutrition. There are so many different schools of thought, so many different paths of education and, ultimately, no definitive answers, so, of course it's going to end up an industry at war.

The problem is that you, as the clients, are the ones who get caught in the crossfire.

A specific teacher will hold a certain belief system regarding their subjects and this will be translated into their teaching in the classroom. As a result, as a coach, you are taught what the teacher holds true at the time. Herein lies the route to the mass confusion within the industry.

The ideals being promoted to you, the client, today as being the *"best* way to lose weight" will probably be debunked by those very same coaches next year. What you have been led to believe in the past by your trainer or nutrition coach will, more than likely, be contradicted by something else they tell you next month. No matter what you are advised to eat, there will be another coach waiting in the wings to inform you that it's toxic or harmful in some way. This isn't me having a dig at coaches out there—not at all, there are many brilliant educators out there who genuinely want to help and who keep their mind open for change. But there are some who can get so caught up in their own paradigms and beliefs that, sometimes, without realizing it, they have a hand in creating *more* anxieties and even encouraging disordered behaviors in clients as a result, and that is certainly helpful to no one.

Surprisingly, for such an important job, a job that is focused entirely on people's health and well-being, there is an awful lot of guess work involved! Unfortunately, this has provided an ideal opportunity for the less ethical coaches and companies out there to promote health products with benefits that are unproven. Is it any surprise that there have been calls for the industry to be regulated? As it stands at the moment, near enough *anyone* can set themselves up as a wellness, nutrition or health coach. This is one of the reasons why we are seeing such an influx of meal replacement diets with the reps who are selling them advertising themselves as nutrition or wellness coaches. More often than not, these reps have not done a single day's official nutrition training, but the fact that they can call themselves 'nutritionist coaches' immediately gives them credibility in the eyes of the public, who know no better than to trust this title. Whereas in truth, these 'coaches' and the companies that provide these meal replacement diet plans are very often more interested in profit than health. The plans are sold to the reps as a business venture and are often part of multi-level marketing systems.

## 18

# Blind Faith

The effect of someone's passion blurring into obsession can be seen within many areas of life. Religious passion can lead to violence and war. Sporting passion leads to team feuds, performance-enhancing drug abuse and fan-based violence. Now, an invigorating passion for nutrition and fitness is leading to fraud, debilitating anxieties and sickness. What makes it harder to escape from in this industry is that this passion for health is actively encouraged in most places you go.

*Now, a disclaimer again here—it is of course extremely important for people to prioritize their own health and take responsibility for their own well-being; naturally, this should always be applauded.*

The problem is that the line between what is a healthy interest in general well-being and a crippling obsession stemming from a desire to appearance-fix is becoming extremely blurred. In the past when the line was crossed, with the act of cutting out food groups or showing anxieties around food or perhaps becoming obsessed with training, it would have been noted and flagged up fairly quickly. These days, however, when these behaviors show up, they are often encouraged and can be met with solid signs of approval. How on earth will you ever know that you are slipping down that slippery slope if every day you drag yourself into the gym, energy lacking, looking thinner and thinner with your mental state declining, you are met with a high-five from a coach saying, "Hey, you're lookin' good! Keep up the good work, girl. You're inspiring!"

One of the popular phrases that is bandied about within the industry is "obsessed is just a word that lazy people use to describe the dedicated." In my opinion (having come out the other side), when I hear this statement now I always just feel that it smacks a little of elitism, with an air of moral superiority. During my dark days, it was one of the statements that I had uppermost in my mind, one I used to tweet and Facebook often. It was this I thought of when I was scowling at my friends for drinking a diet coke (one of the foods on my 'bad' list) or each time I'd shy away from a family dinner to eat my pre-prepared meal or when I'd feel completely worn out and wrecked, but still force myself to get up and train at 6 a.m.

It's strange how this air of arrogance only comes to the fore when our hobby includes diet or fitness-related obsession. You don't see those who have a deep passion for photography, fishing or writing calling out other people as lazy because they don't share their same passion. You don't see nurses hashtagging on Twitter about their *#dedication* to saving lives or farmers posting Facebook statuses about their *#sacrifice* of getting up at 4 a.m. to go plow their field or a pilot insinuating that anyone who can't also fly a plane is just lazy and dumb, so why is it so accepted for fitpros to roll around these social media sites acting as if they are heroes for pre-prepping a week's worth of meals, or some kind of world-class legends for being able to squat properly?

It's about time that the industry humbled itself a little and accepted that all of these things—the training, the *#fitfam* lifestyle, the dieting—they are all just hobbies at the end of the day. Most people have hobbies; it's just that most people don't need to heckle and berate others for not having the same one as them. It's only fitness that seems to see this type of bragging and shaming directed towards those who just simply don't share that same passion.

I remember one time I witnessed a coach talking to a client who happened to be a nurse, a lovely, caring, hard-working nurse based in the local intensive care unit. She was standing next to the scales preparing for her weigh-in with this coach, practically in tears, her face crumpled with fear as she explained to him that she had been unable to go to the gym much that previous week, obviously worried about the prospect of having gained a pound or two. The attitude of her 'coach' in response was sickening. He displayed such an air of superiority as he looked down his nose at her and sneered, "Well, if you wanted it badly enough, you'd make the time. No excuses! No time for that." The most heartbreaking thing about the story is that she just took it. She didn't have the confidence to say that she'd been spending her days saving lives and making sure that people on the verge of death were able to go home and see their families again. She didn't stand up to him and explain that her life was worth so much more than how much time she'd spent at the gym that week. Having watched the interaction as it played out, it made me embarrassed for the industry.

So many kudos are given to physiques and it goes above and beyond anything else in some coaches' minds. This guy acted in a way that showed he felt he was inherently superior to this woman, perhaps because she didn't live up to his physical expectations or maybe she didn't share the same passion that he did, whatever it was. He was suffering from delusions if he felt his physique-based ideals trumped her life-saving ones. Unfortunately, and I mean truly unfortunately, narcissism is a common trait among coaches. It's a character trait that I have witnessed all too many times in those who are meant to be providing a positive, mentally encouraging influence on people, but who instead demean, shame and ridicule.

The rise of social media has given us an ideal platform for this admiration of physique without substance. While it has contributed many positive things, the Internet's growth has also given rise to an enormous increase in deception and fraud—an email address and a few enhanced, posed photos are all you need to fabricate an entire online business profile (and life!). It's important to recognize that Instagram, Twitter, Facebook and other such social media sites are not reserved for the saints of this world. You don't have to show a squeaky clean record to sign up for these sites and, as a result, they provide a stage that gives potential fraudsters and opportunity seekers a chance for grand-scale deception.

Over the last few years, there has been a surge in the number of 'wellness warriors.' These tend to be young attractive women who will go all-out to create online empires based around certain holistic healing protocols, diets or supplements. They have the make-up and the hair and the big-teeth smile, all immaculately posed for each Instagram post they post. From their online presence, we assume that they're as happy as a cat under a leaky cow and also, dangerously, that they are totally trustworthy and have our well-being at heart. Some of these wellness warriors are known for actively boycotting conventional medicine on the basis that they suggest it's not needed, instead encouraging their followers to beat disease naturally with whole foods. Now, I'm not going to let this turn into a debate on whether or not we can heal disease via any way other than traditional medicine, as I keep a very open mind to many alternative forms of therapy, so let's not get pedantic. But to openly encourage thousands or even millions of people to ignore prescribed medical treatment and instead eat, drink or supplement a certain way to beat an established illness is nothing more than totally irresponsible and downright dangerous. We cannot control who sees these social media messages and it is impossible to know who will end up reading them. As a result, this advice has the potential to seep behind the scenes and wreck lives without anyone even knowing about it.

Take a social media site, a pretty face and access to the Internet and, soon enough, you have the chance to build up an army of fanatical followers who will place you on a pedestal and believe everything you say. It only takes a few weeks before these self-made gurus are influencing thousands of people on the choices they make surrounding their diets or exercise routine and influencing people on how to live their lives.

Within just few months, they have acquired the halo of inspiration based on nothing but an attractive face, some cleverly worded posts and blind faith. You base your trust on hearsay or because you saw your friend re-tweet something of hers. Then, after taking everything that these social media 'entrepreneurs' say as gospel, it never fails to amaze me that people get so shocked and surprised when the truth finally comes out about them having absolutely no qualifications, substance or, even worse, when it's discovered that the whole profile was based on lies and fabrication.

This takes on a far more sinister twist when the guru is not just using these platforms to sell the dream of a smaller body size, but to sell the dream of staying alive. One of the best, and at the same time worst, examples of this type of deception by one of these 'wellness warriors' was highlighted recently. A woman had built up an enormous social media empire based upon claims that she was curing her own terminal brain cancer via her diet. She had convinced people that she was getting better on the back of what she was eating. She went on to sell recipe apps, workshops and cookbooks off the back of these claims and amassed a small fortune as a result. She had a fan base into the millions, many of whom were sick themselves and were holding this woman up as their hero, prepared to follow her lead and refuse traditional medicine. So of course, everyone was devastated when eventually it became apparent that she'd fabricated the entire story. Nothing of her story was true and eventually she admitted that she'd never even had cancer.

The painful truth that we have to take on board here is that it's partly our fault. We so love to ogle the body, we so love to feel inspired by the miracle healing diets, and we applaud the healthy lifestyle that these gurus make look like a fairy-tale. They become like the adult versions of the princess characters we idolized as children. We *want* to be told that this perfection of body, this level of health and this idyllic life is possible with relatively little effort. We want to be told that there is a way that we can be that happy too. We are prepared to accept that if we just follow their advice, that could be us soon. We believe that the pictures that they present to us are evidence that a better body will give us a better life and that all we have to do to achieve it is to copy what they do. Sadly though, if you knew the whole truth behind some of these 'inspirational' stories, you'd think twice before blindly giving them your trust and holding their ideas as gospel. If you were to gain access to the whole not-as-pretty truth behind the scenes, you might even step back, look at yourself and begin to realize that you aren't so bad after all. The reality behind these inspirational and ideal lives is often a person full of angst, anxiety and just as many worries as anyone else. These posed selfies, the seeming spontaneous pictures and motivational messages can often be another cover-up for their own deep-rooted insecurities. Of course, the people behind these inspirational profiles will never tell you how they really feel, because they have a reputation to manage, one that is purely validated by others and is meticulously engineered and controlled behind the scenes.

We will never really get the chance to *know* if someone is healthy, happy, sick or obsessed in these situations. We simply have to trust that they're being truthful with the image that they present. So it's not your fault if/when you fall into one of these traps. You weren't to know that your decision to follow a certain diet, workout or health-healing diet protocol was based on fabrication and false information. You trusted that the source was reliable and probably still thought at the time that the industry which describes itself as being responsible for your health and wellness was regulated to stop these kinds of things from happening. Unfortunately, as you now know, it's not.

# 19

# Slim Doesn't Mean Healthy

The majority of people don't tend to want to admit that they are obsessed with looks, especially those I mentioned above, the wellness warriors and social media gurus. They base their image on health over looks, which gives them an 'out' when confronted about contributing to the pressure to conform to body ideal. If they say it's about health, who can argue? In this industry that is full of looks-based obsessions, there is very often a counter-argument—the health thing—ready to go. People buy into this "it's about health" argument as it's natural to assume that certain body shapes—lean and ripped—naturally equal health. However, this is based more on wishful thinking than logic and is a completely flawed argument that needs to be hit head-on. A slim physique absolutely in no way equals health. It is stupid and dangerous to try and assume anyone's level of health from how they look on the outside.

Let's first define what health actually means, as I fear that many in the diet and fitness industry have all but forgotten what it is that we are actually trying to achieve when we talk about health.

Described by the World Health Organization (WHO), "Health is a state of complete physical, mental and social well-being and not merely the absence of disease or infirmity."

Note the combination of the three? Achieving a toned, ripped physique does not give you a free pass to therefore ignore the mental and social well-being needed for health. In fact, here would be a good time to talk about the many cases I have seen in which the achievement of ultimate leanness is actively detrimental to overall health—especially, and much more so, in women. Daniel Meek, a coach and colleague of mine, made it his mission to achieve this ultimate level of leanness for his own experimentation. When asked about the experiences he went through on his journey to achieving this, he said:

> I feel that going through the journey definitely made me a better coach—but only because I knew what was required and could tell clients just how *bad* it was to do. I had the experience of zero sex drive, no energy, no life, no enjoyment.
>
> I feel a bit shallow saying that I am proud of the condition I got into because it took a lot of sacrifice and willpower. It was very hard.
>
> But the key things I stress to every client who wants to go to these levels is that it is not healthy, it is not sustainable and it is definitely NOT going to make you happy. If you are doing it for those reasons, you picked the wrong goal.
>
> I will always coach health first, and I will always ensure my clients know that dieting to get very lean is not healthy— I think you just have to be honest and educate clients from your experience.
>
> After my shoot I went back to enjoying food, not tracking and having a life. All of which I am extremely grateful for and now don't take for granted!

As bad as it can get for a guy, for a woman to achieve these levels of leanness we see in the images, fitspiration memes and media campaigns will be even harder and may result in far worse side-effects than a man experiences. On top of the sexual dysfunction, the general feelings of stress, restriction and obsession, you can also add hormone dysregulation and mood disorders to the list.

Getting into and sustaining the lifestyle that is required to achieve these 'photo shoot' levels of physique is not, in any shape or form, a bed of roses. Even those who do achieve this level of leanness often do not stay that way all year round.

This works both ways, as similar logic applies to a person

who may be walking around 10 kilos (22 pounds) above 'optimal' weight, but if they are otherwise healthy, mentally and emotionally, they are likely to be in better health, or similar health at least, than a slim but depressed, anxious and socially isolated person of the same age.

We don't want to risk looking superficial, so we have found what many believe to be the perfect counter-argument of 'health' that gives an acceptable excuse to body shame. The crux of this matter is that you cannot, no matter who you are, tell a person's health by looking at their outside physique. We have created a society where this is thought to be possible, simply because we need an excuse to judge ourselves and others on how we look in swimwear. It's time that it stopped as, far too often, this assumption is doing far more harm than good.

I'll give you a real-life example of the devastating effects that this type of physique-based assumption of health can have. A few years back, I was working in a local gym where I met a girl. A young, quiet girl who joined because she wanted to lose a few pounds for a holiday. She started to come in a few times a week, lasting for a few months. She achieved what she'd set out to achieve in losing a few pounds, plus a little more. So of course, in response to this, people had started to notice. First came the comments about how great she looked and how she should "keep up the good work!" This attention grew just as quick as she shrank. It sparked something in her, this attention she was getting. However, the comments were often marred with state-ments such as "Keep going" and "You're almost there!" and these made her feel like she still had further to go. She described to me some time later that her thoughts as a result of these comments were "Why are people saying 'keep going'? I must still look fat." So, soon she was spending two hours a day, every day, in the gym. She dropped more and more weight, and yes, the compli-ments kept on coming. Strangers would be approaching her to tell her how inspiring she was and how amazing she looked and, again, advising her to keep up this great work.

Unfortunately, what they didn't realize was that within the space of a year, this once lively and bubbly young girl's quest to lose a few pounds for a holiday had since developed into severe bulimia. She was eating barely 500 kilocalories a day, followed up with regular binging sessions followed by purging. She'd be spending two weary hours on the cardio equipment every day, and people were in absolute awe. Women flocked to the instructors to ask what she was doing to lose so much weight and asking if they could possibly divulge her training program so they could follow the same one.

Inside, this girl was in bits emotionally and severely physically ill. Yet, these assumptions about her health in relation to her looks and the praise from the people around her were actively encouraging her to carry on and push for more.

Further down the road, once she was in recovery, she became a client of mine. I had been able to tell something was amiss after I'd approached her and we'd started chatting. She explained how a family member had picked up on the problem and she'd agreed to start treatment for the disorder. Eventually, we started to work together in the gym to help build her muscular strength, and confidence, back up.

The treatment was successful. She gained some weight back and she was rebuilding her muscle strength and recovering extremely well. Until one day when a male gym member approached her, not knowing her from Adam. He decided to take it upon himself to advise her that she should "be careful as she was putting the weight back on."

Now, I know as much as you do that we cannot control other people. We have no way of controlling what comes out of the mouths of the folks around us. Nor should we, as freedom of speech is precious in this world. Still, I feel it's about time that we begin to recognize when freedom of speech is just an excuse to be an ass to another person, because we have somehow accepted that it's absolutely okay to comment on other people's weight without knowing the story behind the person. This is not okay. His filter was disengaged and he went ahead and said something that there was absolutely no need for him, or anyone else, to say. This one remark, brought on by a stranger's assumption based on her looks, had the potential to slam this girl straight back into that dark and dangerous place that once threatened her life.

We have got to stop this assumption that it's okay to judge and comment on people's appearance without regard for the effect our words may have.

Luckily, this girl kept her resolve and made the adult decision to ignore it. However, a week or so later, after a second comment by someone else in the same gym—yes, it happened twice—that was said "in jest" about her "filling out again," she felt she was forced into a situation of having to publicly defend herself, giving her no option but to openly admit she was in recovery from bulimia and in fact this 'filling out' was necessary for her to *live*. This situation is simply unacceptable; she should never have been forced into disclosing such personal information just to defend changes on the outside of her body to strangers. As a society, we have made it perfectly fine to discuss other people's weight freely; therefore we have created this monster of pressure that we, ourselves, have to deal with. Yet, as witnessed so many times, we still react with shock and horror when this accepted open door of judgment starts to affect us or our families personally.

The diet and fitness industry often uses the power behind this pressure as it continues to make money from it. Instead of giving help to the girls who are riddled with insecurities, self-hate and crippling obsessions, we encourage them to diet harder and give trophies for it. We feed the obsession and then we wonder why it is that eating disorders are on the rise within our primary schools.

The situation we find ourselves in as a result of this body-beautiful obsession is that, in many cases, those suffering with illnesses and health battles are being met with praise because of the effect that the illnesses have on their looks. Being complimented for looking 'better' while being in the throes of a devastating illness and criticized when in recovery, all stemming from the effects on body weight, is becoming more and more common.

Here are just a few real-world examples of this that I have come across recently:

I have colitis and experienced people telling me how good I looked when I was drastically sick and then felt guilty (but more so largely happy) when I started gaining weight…

I'd like to be thinner, but my mental well-being takes precedence. I have to let go of all of those memories of people complimenting me on how great I looked when I was obviously sick and painfully thin. I had to let go of how pious I felt when I was eating 'right.'

Yeah. When I was dying of anorexia, people told me how beautiful I looked. But when I recovered from that and gained weight and was at the weight the doctors wanted me, I got told that I'm fat and ugly.

We have got to stop worshiping protruding hip bones, without understanding what the owner has done to get them. We have mothers who would be devastated at the knowledge that their teenage daughter is making herself sick after eating, or crying herself to sleep every night because she doesn't look like the models on Instagram, but how can we expect anything different when at the same time that same mother is reading "How To Get Skinny in Six Weeks" articles, cutting out entire food groups and constantly talking about other women's weight? Minds—young or old—are not immune to this information. These subconscious messages that looks equal worthiness will be picked up, stored and regurgitated for the rest of her life. We cannot get angry and sad when we hear of a ten-year-old child in the grips of anorexia when the language, behavior and  teachings around her all point to weight and body shape being so important.

On a social media platform recently, I saw some before-and-after weight-loss pictures of a girl who must have been no older than 11 years old, with accompanying messages about how well the diet is working that she was on. As I looked through the list of comments on the post, it was, shockingly, full of admiration and praise about how much 'better' this young girl had become now that she'd lost some weight. The damage something like this can have can be devastating, setting this girl up for a life where her subconscious mind tells her that to have a slimmer body means to be praised, loved and even accepted by strangers.

# When Inspiration Isn't Inspiring

If you've been around the social media sphere for the past few years, then you'll most likely have heard the word 'fitspiration' and will have witnessed the type of images that accompany this label. The idea forms from pictures of physiques, often with quotes over the top, which are supposedly motivation to get fit— fitspiration being the play on words to describe inspiration in line with fitness.

The images are extreme and, more often than not, show digitally enhanced physiques which are presented with a statement such as "You can feel sore tomorrow or you can feel sorry tomorrow" or a similar sort of 'threat' or guilt-inducing message for those who don't yet match up to this fitness body ideal. These types of images play the shame card, resulting in feelings of guilt and failure. They leave you questioning your lifestyle, while giving you the message that if you go and beat yourself up in the gym today, you'll wake up happy tomorrow. This 'motivational' movement is once again selling you the dream of *the* body, which you associate with the dream life.

Given there is no rational basis behind any of these images, I feel stupid for even suggesting there may be—there is none. In any case, they contradict each other hugely. For example, one has the caption "Suck it up now and you won't have to suck it in later" above an image of a girl with a tiny waist, visible abs on show, drinking from a bottle of water—giving you the impression that all you have to do is drink more water and you will stand a chance of achieving this level of physique. Off you go, chug, chug, chug, expecting results similar to Popeye eating his spinach. However, then you stumble across another one that talks about how it takes years of blood, sweat and tears to get fit, while informing you that you are never allowed to quit! Hmm.

I just wanted to highlight one of the hundreds of contradictions that you are exposed to with these memes. To be honest, it is a fruitless task to try and find any solid and common sense behind any of these fitspiration images. They weren't created for any other purpose than to shame and induce guilt. Fitspiration often depicts the moral status of working out being on par with saving the world with your own bare hands. Some of them are quite comical, but you have to be able to see past the shame to appreciate the humor. It's deranged to assume that these pictures were created with any worry over integrity—they use photoshopped images, for goodness' sake, effectively trying to make you feel guilty for being *real*.

Let's look further at social media as it has such an almighty impact on everything we are talking about. In fact, a study has shown that the media (43.5%), advertising (16.8%) and celebrity culture (12.5%) together account for almost *three quarters* of the influence on body image in society.

On Instagram alone, you will find over 5 million images with a fitspiration hashtag. These images get shared on social media platforms all over the world, every day. Some women I have spoken to even use these images as screensavers to encourage their food restriction on days they feel hungry!

Which brings me to 'thinspiration.' This is a term that you may have heard of similar to 'fitspiration,' but rather than the pursuit of fitness, these images are dedicated to the pursuit of extreme thinness. These images are connected to a movement that is known as 'pro-ana' which is short for pro-anorexia, referring to the promotion of behaviors related to the eating disorder, while suggesting that anorexia is a lifestyle choice as opposed to an illness.

Many of these images feature emaciated girls, sometimes on the verge of death, with similar types of quotes or sayings, usually encouraging fellow sufferers to push further, restrict more, embrace their hunger and do anything to succeed in starving their way to 'perfection.'

The harsh truth is that the images used in our industry's beloved fitspiration movement are not all that different to those used by the thinspiration sites and a recent study was done to highlight this. The researchers looked at fifty of each category of site, and compared the images and content. They found the following:

Thinspiration sites featured more content related to losing weight or fat, praising thinness, showing a thin pose and providing food guilt messages than Fitspiration sites. However, sites did not differ on guilt-inducing messages regarding weight or the body, fat/weight stigmatization, the presence of objectifying phrases, and dieting/restraint messages. Overall, 88% of Thinspiration sites and 80% of Fitspiration sites contained one or more of the coded variables…

Many of the social media platforms that share these fitspiration images and slogans can so often yank out the health card as soon as they are challenged, just like we spoke about earlier. They are often positioning themselves to be advocates of health and wellness, defending their decision to promote and share these images as they suggest they are doing so from a health and motivational standpoint.

However, unfortunately, just how can they attest to a photo showing optimal health, unless they personally know the person in every single one of these fitspirational pictures? Which I am highly sure they do not. Harriet Williamson, a writer and journalist, has a strong opinion on this subject and did her own investigation to prove just how ridiculous this defense line of advocating health is. Harriet, thankfully, is now in recovery from anorexia, but during the years of being in the grips of her illness, she used to be a frequent visitor to these pro-ana sites. Here, she explains a recent experiment she did to prove that many of these pages, which claim to be sharing fitspiration images on the basis of health advocacy, are nothing more than 'thinspiration' pages in disguise.

A popular Tumblr account that describes itself as 'healthy fitspiration' and 'body positive' is paradoxically filled with near-emaciated bodies and one of them is mine, which I submitted as a test. My body is permanently damaged by anorexia and I am medically advised against any exercise other than brisk walking. The idea that 'fitspo' images have anything to do with health or fitness is entirely spurious and the use of my picture is proof of this. Thin does not necessarily mean healthy and neither does it mean fit.

The fitspiration images are continually accepted into the health and fitness industry and thus, society, because they are promoted as positive motivation. If you question such images, you can often be met with extreme defensiveness, followed by an explanation that they are "encouraging people to push for more and become better," whatever 'better' means. However, the psychology behind these messages tends to disagree. We can understand this further by looking at the different types of motivation that we tend to work from—intrinsic and extrinsic. Intrinsic motivation is when you take part in something for the enjoyment of it, for example taking part in a football match simply for the enjoyment of playing the game, whereas to be extrinsically motivated would mean you are playing purely to win. Extrinsic motivation promises reward for your efforts, whereas with intrinsic, the reward is in the taking part. Extrinsic motivation can also come from external praise, such as being supported or encouraged by family or even a physician.

Psychologists agree that a combination of the two within our lives can be a good thing. However, embarking on a fitness regime or diet plan purely for extrinsic reasons shows that it is not likely to be sustained for long. Extrinsic motivation will not provide the push needed to get past common hurdles such as boredom or being busy; basically, extrinsically motivated programs will see you more likely to give up when challenged or faced with obstacles.

Some behavior experts consider appearance to be extrinsic in nature, so the trouble with fitspiration, and the body-shaming tactics that some less scrupulous coaches have decided to adopt, is that they can actually exacerbate issues. These images encourage the pursuit of fitness purely on the basis of the perceived reward of this ideal physique, as opposed to encouraging the actual enjoyment of exercise, while prioritizing the pursuit of health and well-being—which is definitely not defined by your looks.

Time and time again, shaming people into embarking on diets or exercise programs has been shown not to be an effective way to create long-term behavior change.

A recent study found that those who *think* they are overweight (even when they aren't) are more likely to actually gain weight in the future as a response. The researchers said:

Perceiving oneself as being 'overweight' is counter-intuitively associated with an increased risk of future weight gain among US and UK adults. They found a link between the stress of thinking themselves as being overweight, to the actual overeating that caused this fear to become true…perceiving oneself as being overweight was associated with overeating in response to stress and this mediated the relationship between perceived overweight and weight gain.

The researchers also suggested that a reason for this could be that those who think of themselves as overweight are more likely to embark on crash diets which, in turn, are then more likely to see future rebound weight gain.

I can anecdotally back this up myself. The poorer the body image that a client has shown, the more likely we are to see vast fluctuations in actual weight. When weight becomes so important in achieving self-worth and a person 'feels' that they are overweight, even when they are not, it is very likely that they will undertake diets, excessive exercise and short-term 'programs' that tick all the boxes—extreme, unsustainable and misery-inducing.

Body-shaming has become a 'thing' thanks to a handful of 'celebrities' who have adopted the tough-love approach, thinking that they are doing the right thing to help those who are overweight, whereas in fact, I think honestly it's just a sick method of entertainment that they seem to get away with because of, oh, guess what? They play the health card!

The problem is that this new form of 'motivation' can be directed at anyone, 'overweight' (unless diagnosed in a clinical setting) can be entirely subjective in a person's mind, and these harsh, unforgiving messages directed towards overweight people are also likely to be picked up by those who aren't overweight. Those who have a poor body image will view themselves in this overweight category—and if they then choose to embark on a crash diet in response to the shaming they have been exposed to, it may even mean that they *become* overweight in the future as a result. So, not only is body-shaming not part of the solution as these partakers suggest, it's actually more likely to be an active part of the problem.

Brené Brown, PhD, a shame and vulnerability researcher, has also found an inverse relationship between shame and the belief that one is capable of long-term behavior change. She has found that shame often leads to more shame, explaining: "as a person is exposed to shame, it can lead to further destructive behaviors that result in more shame, a vicious cycle."

Jane Wardle, director of the Cancer Research UK Health Behaviour Centre at University College London, said in a statement in response to their study that also showed weight discrimination to be part of the problem, not the solution: "Everyone, including doctors, should stop blaming and shaming people for their weight and offer support, and where appropriate, treatment."

The more we learn about the psychology and behaviors behind weight, body image and self-esteem, the more it becomes glaringly obvious that shaming and judging only serve to make the problems we have discussed worse. It doesn't help those who do genuinely want or need to lose weight, and it may actually encourage those at a healthy weight, but with poor body image, to engage in behaviors that result in increased risk of health problems in the future.

There is also another issue that these fitspiration images present to us. An elephant is in the room, hiding the small but significant fact that the images we are discussing often aren't even *real*. The digital enhancing process that the media use as the norm these days is becoming a problem. Photoshopping is a topic that everyone knows about, but no one really seems to want to do anything about. When I talk about how much these 'motivational' images are altered—smoothed, slimmed and tightened—it's often met with a response of "Yeah, but it happens everywhere—we should just get used to it!"

To an extent, I understand that to try and encourage companies to stop altering images would be a fruitless task, but my issue is that these images are the very ones that are being paraded around as the ideal physique, which is contributing hugely to the body image crisis we have in the world right now.

Change can occur, but first, we have to at least decide that we want it and, second, we have to understand that the biggest and most effective route of change needs to occur within our own minds. We can control what we think and how we respond to things; therefore it is up to each individual to prioritize self-esteem and self-love enough to result in these images, and the pressure to conform as a response, losing their power against us.

If you walk into any newsagent or store and take a look at the magazine selection tailored to women, I would challenge you to find any without reference to weight, dieting or body shape on the front cover (unless you are looking at *Horse & Hound*, and even then I wouldn't be so sure). Trying to get the magazine companies to change this would be pointless, because currently, these things sell. However, there is one simple thing that you can do here to immediately make a difference to how *you* feel and that is to simply opt out of buying these publications. Save yourself the time and value your mind a bit more. The media and advertising account for almost three-quarters of the influence on our body image in society, so when we have teenage girls (or women of any age!) reading articles about "dropping 10 kg" to look hot on one page, while being encouraged to "feel confident in your own skin!" on the next, then turning over to see "shocking" celeb weight gain or cellulite pics on the page after that, it becomes an insult to our intelligence and only serves to confuse, contradict and control us.

Before a few years ago, these digital enhancing techniques were limited to the small selection of magazines from the top media companies. Even though it was still wrong to present what are essentially false images to the public as real, we could cope as we knew that they were limited to the covers of magazines and the billboards on the streets, and even then, the digital enhancing wasn't at the level that we are exposed to now. However, that has changed with the advance of technology over the past ten years. Now, household computers have editing software as standard that can alter and enhance your summer holiday snaps to embody ultimate catwalk perfection. We have smartphone apps at our fingertips that can edit blemishes away from selfies in seconds. Filters are used as standard and, as a result, barely any photographs you see on social media these days are 100% raw and untouched.

It is messing with our minds as we are now viewing these altered images as normal and subconsciously viewing the enhanced bodies in them as 'average' when they are absolutely nothing of the sort. Because we never see the body behind the edits in real life, we begin to assume that it's just us who doesn't fit that mold of perfection that, seemingly from the photos, everyone else does.

The contradictory habits of these magazines can be highlighted in nearly every issue if you look. There have been examples of magazine covers featuring an interview with a famous figure about her struggle with an eating disorder, with another headline below entitled "How to get an insane body! It'll hurt, but you'll look hot!"

Or another example was a publication which featured an issue dedicated to "Body Confidence," using a celebrity who openly expressed her own body confidence battles, but the magazine decided to still go ahead and photoshop her images for the feature.

As a result of technological advances, these enhancements are getting far trickier to police. We have women down at the local gym who are using these editing apps to become more defined, tanned or toned in their Facebook profile. Perhaps more worryingly, schoolyards are becoming the new stage for filtered selfies. We have ended up in a society where people are becoming more and more desperately unhappy about how they look. Seventy-eight percent of 17-year-old girls are unhappy with their body. By the age of 14, half of girls and one third of boys have been on a diet to try and change their body shape. Fourteen-year-olds are not dieting for health reasons. Teens haven't suddenly developed an interest in fat burners and juice fasts because they want to take care of their body. They are doing it purely to appearance-fix because all they see around them are these images and suggestions as to what it takes to be worthy of love and acceptance, and what it takes, it seems, is packaged up in the body beautiful. The onset of a poor body image is getting younger and younger, and unfortunately it doesn't just diminish as a person gets older. Hating how we look unfortunately is not something that we just grow out of. Once sparked, this sense of unease and unworthiness with who we are will grow and grow and continue building to epic proportions, as it has done with the 10 million women in the UK who report that they feel 'depressed' because of the way they look. If it isn't actively dealt with at the source—our core sense of self-esteem—we will just continue trying to throw money at treating the symptoms, akin to expecting a sticking plaster to help heal a broken bone. More work, more time and more respect needs to be given to the building of our self-esteem, while at the same time moving away from this obsessive need to fix our self-image. David G. Myers, PhD, tells us that "an abundance of empirical research conducted worldwide has revealed that self-esteem is a universal and crucial factor that is related to the level of happiness amongst people." Since, throughout my many years of epiphanies and research, happiness seems to be what everyone is trying to find, it makes sense to start there.

# 21

# Happy People Like Themselves

A large part of this upcoming process will be aimed at releasing the long-held negative beliefs from your subconscious mind that tell you that you can't be happy until you look 'better' or that you 'need' to lose weight before you can go on holiday—or go for that promotion or leave your husband or buy a new dress—or whatever it is that you believe your weight (or how you look) is stopping you from doing. We also need to go deeper than these, because all of these beliefs start with the same thought process. The same thought process that has you believe that you need to look like the Instagram models in order to be accepted by others or to be able to accept yourself.

Your subconscious mind rules your decisions, actions and behaviors 95% of the time. It is this part of your brain that will be in charge of how you feel on a day-to-day basis. Beliefs are just collections of thought patterns. A thought that we think over and over can quickly become a belief that we hold as fact. If your subconscious stays full of those beliefs we just talked about, the beliefs that you need to change physically in order to be worthy of self-love, then nothing will change within you and nothing will change within your life. It isn't as simple as just 'thinking differently'; it takes time, commitment and effort to change your subconscious beliefs. The great thing is that after this work and effort, you will genuinely feel a massive shift within your life—no invisible pots of gold at the end of an expensive rainbow—because once you commit to changing your thoughts, you really will change your life.

You may understand and appreciate everything that I've written so far, but if we don't follow this information up with action, you'll quickly revert to basing your self-worth on your dress size, which will lead you straight back into this yo-yo cycle that we are pulling you out from.

My aim for you, and all my clients, is to help you to achieve that feeling of being at peace with who you are, with the ability to feel comfortable in your own skin without that constant internal nag that you should/would/could/ought to be someone or something else. Sometimes when we first embark on this mission, I see a bit of concern in-between the initial phases of energy and excitement. I know where these flecks of concern come from. It tends to be because this kind of work—reprogramming your subconscious and working to build unconditional self-love—can sound, to some, a bit 'woo-woo.'

We have been conditioned to ignore every aspect of ourselves apart from what we can physically see and measure. Many have no idea just how significant mindset, psychology and mental health is to our physical health, because they consistently ignore the power of anything that is not visible to their naked eye. Likely because they were brought up to think that way, their childhood teachings didn't include anything about mindset or beliefs, whereas the next person who was brought up to see mental health as just as important as physical will see the benefits of doing this type of work straight away.

There is also another reason that people sometimes turn away from this sort of self-development work. In the past I have experienced some who immediately back off, fearing the work because they know that it's absolutely not a quick fix and that the changes they wish to see will not happen overnight. Deep down, they know that challenging their mindset will be hard work; it's not just a pill to take or a diet plan to follow—it means continuous action, every day. Having to look within and begin to take responsibility for why you are where you are in life, and for how you feel in response to where you are, for many people can just be too much to contemplate.

I have to explain to them that dealing with your feelings,

changing how you respond to things and learning to change your beliefs and expectations, which will therefore change your life, is hard work, and that is precisely why most people don't try. If it was easy, everyone would be doing it. Everyone would be walking around with a solid, consistent and unconditional appreciation for themselves, blind to the pressures around them to conform, living a life they want to live and enjoying the process immensely. Yet it's quite obvious that the majority of people don't do this. Instead, they spend their time and money on fixing the symptoms, which doesn't actually fix anything in the long run—hence the vicious and never-ending cycle.

Right now to you, having not started the process of change yet, it will feel virtually impossible to imagine being able to love who you are, as you are. It will feel overwhelming to think about looking in the mirror and appreciating, as opposed to scrutinizing, your body, and it will feel incomprehensible to imagine yourself never feeling unworthy again. But I assure you, it will soon feel natural and right.

Well, we are about to start the journey towards this life, but I want you to know that there may be times you get tempted to turn back. Often it's far easier to swivel on your heels and re-join the ingrained routine back down at the local diet club than it is to have to take on the task of this life-changing mindset work. Even so, I want you to think about the long game. What will happen if you don't do this? Where will you be in ten years if you close this book now and never return to it again? You have a chance at your fingertips to make significant, powerful and long-lasting changes within your life—the only decision you have to make is whether you use it.

## 22

# Letting Go of the Dream

What I've come to expect from my time in this world is that there will always be those who want to prove their point, while proving others wrong. From being in the position of stepping out, going against the grain of the normality and having to put views forward that have previously been thought of as unimportant and sometimes even taboo, I have always been aware that I will likely come up against some stick. People will always, naturally, defend their own paradigms; it's just human nature. I fully expect to receive letters telling me how a sugar-free, gluten-free, meat-free diet was the key to a person's ultimate life-affirming happiness, or that a 10 kilo weight loss resulted in an abundance of confidence and internal peace greater than any mindset work could ever achieve. There will be people around you that tell *you* similar things, too. All I will say is this—there is no need to defend, argue or prove wrong. Don't get dragged into a 'my way is the right way' conversation, as, quite frankly, that is the exact situation I am trying to rid the world of! My aim is to see a world full of women who feel absolutely awesome in their own skin, with an abundance of unconditional self-love. I have no interest in proving anyone wrong. Remember, I always wanted to know that weight loss had the ability to create happiness. After all, that's what I spent so much of my own life trying to prove! Even so, when I was so often seeing the opposite, I just simply had to admit defeat. If someone loses weight and seems to be living proof that weight loss alone does result in authentic self-love for the rest of their life (not just for a month or two), then please, congratulate them. A true indication as to whether they are being authentic or not is to observe how they speak to you. When people are truly happy within themselves, they will find no need to disrespect what you are choosing to do; they will simply encourage and support you in doing what helps you. As the saying goes, "Hurt people hurt people." A sure-fire way to know if someone is as happy and confident as they say they are is to notice how they treat you. They'll show you the proof of their own self-love via their words and actions to others.

In situations where you think you are seeing real-world evidence of weight loss breeding true happiness—before diving back onto the bandwagon—I'd also ask you to look for further evidence before taking it all at face value. What else changed in their life at the same time as the weight loss? Was it just weight loss in isolation that made the difference or did their life change in other ways at the same time? Was it the weight loss or was it the mindset change? Finally, remember—the best yardstick for success in these situations is simply time gone by. For a true 'diet success,' we need to see evidence that the weight loss has been maintained, as well as the self-love, confidence and emotional health five years down the line.

If you come up against anyone who tries to put a damper on what you are doing, which you likely will as people don't tend to like what they don't understand, there is no need to justify anything. That isn't your job. Just nod and accept that they are still on their own journey. Remember, you once most likely would have agreed with their opinion had you been introduced to the idea before you were ready. Their time will come, but that makes no odds to you right now, so focus on your own life, your own journey and let them focus on theirs.

*NB: If this person persists to the point of making you uncomfortable, then it may be time to re-evaluate the amount of time you spend in their company. Fear not, Part Three of the book will help you here.*

The work coming up in this book is designed for those of you who are stuck in that yo-yo diet cycle because you buy into the belief that a smaller dress size is the route to self-love. This is not a book designed to convince you that you should never attempt to lose weight. What you may find is that once you prioritize the inner work—the self-esteem building and fulfillment finding—your physical body will have more of a chance to take care of itself naturally, without the internal complications, yo-yo-ing, and emotional eating or restricting. Still, this shouldn't be the reason you embark on these tasks ahead. The outcome I want for you is to feel worthy of acceptance, right now, with no external conditions attached. So, what you are doing is accepting that right now, weight loss isn't the priority.

By now I hope you are starting to understand that weight loss/gain or weight-controlling behaviors such as emotional eating or restrictive eating are symptoms of your internal emotional and mental state. What you need to prioritize first is finding compassion for yourself and focusing on self-love. Once you are on this track, your physical priorities will become more a job of *health* maintenance, rather than appearance-fixing, as you will have the ability to see your body size and shape as totally individual and separate from how worthy of love and acceptance you are.

Once you have experienced this unconditional self-love, your confidence, self-esteem and happiness will stay consistent. No matter who you are with, no matter what you weigh and no matter what situation you find yourself in, you will be able to show up to any given situation and feel good enough and worthy enough to be there as your true and authentic self, with no voice inside telling you that you should be thinner or leaner or a better dieter.

So before we move on, I want to ask how you are feeling having come to the end of this first section. Take some time for all of this to sink in. I'm expecting you to change your opinion of something very indoctrinated, so don't feel bad if you need to take a day or two to mull this first section of information over and get it all straight in your head before moving on.

Once you feel ready to embark on the next step, turn the page and delve into Part Two, where I will begin to explain the reasons why this type of mindset work is the most important part of the journey when it comes to achieving long-term change. Feel excited at this point, because the journey ahead has the potential to be an extremely powerful one.

*Authenticity is the daily practice of letting go of who we think we're supposed to be and embracing who we are.*
—Brené Brown

# Part Two

*To experience true self-love, you have to conquer the fear of your own body.*
—Unknown

In the previous section, we have seen how the dream of experiencing self-love and happiness has been sold to you as something you can achieve via improving or 'fixing' how you look. The reasons you became obsessed with different diets—those initial thought processes that fired up your progressively unhealthy relationship with food, that deep desire to place coaches on a pedestal—have all been born of a belief that the coach or the plan can fix you. Which speaks directly to your desire to change your physical, outer being in order for your internal being to feel worthy of self-love and acceptance.

However, not everyone is obsessed with changing her physical body and it's important to recognize that. Sometimes I speak to people about what I do and what I coach and write about, and they look at me like I'm crazy. In their minds, it's ridiculous to think that a pressure to look better can create such emotional turmoil in some people. They have no idea what it feels like, so cannot comprehend why it's so much of an issue. This is simply because not everyone has learnt to base their feelings of worthiness on how they look. Your early years as you grew up, your teachings from the world around you and the information you sucked into your subconscious mind will determine how you eventually start to perceive your overall worth as a person.

Some will attribute their sense of worth to work-based success—for instance, if someone has learnt that to be busy is to be respected and to be stressed is a social symbol of importance, then they will more likely find that they start to run into issues stemming from overwork, stress, fatigue and quite possibly burnout. Rather than googling different diets, exercises and thumbing over Instagram's clean-eating accounts, they will likely be spending their days finding things to do, taking on extra projects, and generally feeling stressed and exhausted from working so hard, often not even particularly productively. Because they fear that to rest or take time out will mean that they're seen as lazy or unsuccessful.

Another common one is financial success. You may know of some people who feel their worthiness is based upon their bank statements each month, who will also work and work to the point of illness or the neglect of their family, but this time because of the need to see their financial worth increase. Their assets or material possessions correlate directly with how worthy they feel they are in their world.

All of these examples of belief structure are similar at their base level, all responding to a fear of 'lack.' All these result in the same thought process as you when you are spending your days obsessing about the contents of your plate, comparing your butt to those of everyone around you and constantly worrying about the size of your thighs… because this is how *you* see your worth.

Think about this for a second. If you decide that your worth is based on how lean you are, then it will be. If you believe that your worth is decided by how 'clean' you eat, then it will be. Because the only person who determines your worth is you. Therefore, if you change your subconscious and begin to believe that your worth isn't determined by how many times a week you exercise, then it won't be. How you view your worth all boils down to just a simple change of mindset. It's up to you how worthy you feel!

I maintain that our subconscious mind holds all the cards when it comes to how we feel and what we believe about ourselves. If we don't deal with all of this at the root of the problem—by getting into your mind and reprogramming how your subconscious speaks to you—then there is a high chance that these appearance-based self-worth beliefs will just morph into other areas of your life. For example, simply just deciding to stop training when you don't want to, eating with more balance and flexibility and dealing with your obsessive diet behaviors on the surface can feel great in the short term. For a few weeks, you'll feel like you have got to grips with it all and that you are finally free. But if that belief of 'I'm not enough' is still burning away strongly within you, you will soon find something else external that replaces it. Something different will become the answer: how stressed you are, how much work you do, how much money you have, how perfect your children are, who your partner is. Without the deeper mindset work, no sooner than you wake up no longer worrying about what is on your plate, you'll be waking up worrying about what is in your bank account. Rather than you having achieved unconditional self-love, your measurements of your self-worth have just morphed into a different area of your life. It's a common scenario, one that shows us the importance of dealing with these things at the root of the issue.

There will forever be examples of your not-enough-ness presented to you wherever you look. There will always be people out there who are something you are not. Without making these deep-rooted changes to your mindset, it becomes a constant battle as you live life trying to fit yourself into the acceptable category everywhere you go. How exhausting!

Everything we do in life has an emotion at the root of it. The emotion that lay at the root of my own disordered eating behaviors, as well as those of many others, was fear. Fear of rejection, fear of ridicule or criticism—these fears lay at the base of so many of the different behaviors that we have talked about.

# 23

# Standing in the Face of Fear

*Always be yourself, express yourself, have faith in yourself; do not go out and look for a successful personality and duplicate it.*
—Bruce Lee

Fear is often cited as the most common emotion at the root of our lack of worthiness. We get stuck in the cycle of trying to change who we are on the surface because deep down we are terrified of being seen for who we really are underneath. This fear is born because we are convinced that who we really are—the core of us—is unworthy of being accepted by others.

There is a word that we rarely say as it has such negative connotations: *shame*. We tend to feel embarrassed to admit that we've ever felt any sense of shame. It's easier to ignore it and push it to the side so as not to appear weak in any way. But we cannot ignore it at this point, because shame is a huge part of that fear that stands at the root of these issues we are talking about. Shame is the instigator in this ongoing catfight we have taken up within ourselves in order to become 'enough.'

Shame is the food that feeds the fear monster. It is the fuel for our feelings of not being pretty enough, slim enough, rich enough or intelligent enough. It has the power to convince you that it's worth spending as much time as you would in a full-time job trying to cover up what is real, spending your life trying to find a way to 'fix' these areas that the fear monster loves to highlight to you. By striving to be thinner, prettier and funnier, we misguidedly think that we are protecting ourselves from any future negative feelings.

"If I can just become _____ then I'll never be judged. I'll never be hurt. I'll feel worthy and accepted. I can be free!"

Until next time.

In order to stop being ruled by fear-based, protecting behaviors, we need to alter your subconscious thought patterns to become less obsessive about who you aren't and more focused on embracing who you *are*.

This mindset shift lies at the center of you being able to live the rest of your life experiencing a true and authentic confidence, feeling a sense of contentment about yourself.

It is the resulting emotions created by the fear monster that tell you that you need to go on a new diet every week, because the monster convinces you that you will be judged shamefully by everyone you come across if you don't start striving to look better. The monster also tells you that you need to sign up to that new coach you met who was promising the quick transformation for the same reason. Just like it's that dang monster again who whispers that you really ought to feel guilty for not working out every day last week or for eating that biscuit. The fear monster is watching your every move, waiting to pounce.

He judges you more than the rest of the world put together. That judgment that you fear so much from others is strongest within YOU!

When we spend our lives living in this constant state of fear of judgment, it affects everything we do. From this state of being, we can never know who we really are, we can never experience what it would be like to live as our greatest self who has the ability to show up, be seen and create waves in whatever it is that we were put on this earth to do. Instead, we accept a life where we prioritize pleasing others, a life that we are happy to let slip by quietly so as not to disturb or upset anyone. From trying to cover up and hide our greatest strengths in order to make ourselves a carbon copy of what we deem to be acceptable, all we achieve is another life spent feeling exhausted, burnt-out and numb.

We go to great lengths to protect ourselves from the pain of

having acceptance taken away from us, so depending on which 'tribe' we are spending the most time with, we will adopt behaviors and habits that will see us fitting into their environment. Ever noticed how at different stages of your life, you've prioritized different things? I wonder if maybe this obsession with diets and fitness you have now only began when you moved in to a specific neighborhood or part of town, or perhaps when you got a new job? All of these changes in environment would have meant that your 'tribe' changed with it. Maybe it was as soon as your friend started to get into 'clean eating' that you felt you needed to as well in order to keep the friendship alive? Her tribe changed, thus you changed to keep up with that for fear of losing her acceptance.

The circumstances around us will dictate which persona we choose to present to the world. Wherever we go and whoever we see, we take our chameleon masks with us, ready and prepped to change into whatever we think will be accepted by the crowd. We put up the walls around the real us and decide to wear whatever disguise we feel is needed to fit in—which, importantly, is dependent on what we think *they* want to see from us. Which means, of course, that even when we are rejected and judged, we're being rejected for something that we made up, not who we *really* are. This, of course, makes it a lot easier for us to bear.

We'll call this disguised version of you your *false-self*. This is how I will describe the "if I just act like this, I'll be okay—they'll like me" false image you present to the world in certain external situations. When you are barefaced, raw, your true self with no disguise, you are presenting your authentic self and this we will call your *true-self*.

With social media being as powerful and as life-consuming as it is these days, we are far more likely to end up projecting a false-self full time if we are not careful. Before smartphones and tablets, we didn't have opportunities to 'check in' everywhere we went or to provide our friends with an hour-by-hour description of our day. We would have spent much more time without the need for constant, hour-by-hour acceptance. These days, false-self projections have become a full-time requirement for many people, as they live their lives in full view of the thousands of friends, acquaintances and sometimes even strangers that they have on their expanding social media lists. What once would have been our most precious opportunities to rest and spend time as our true-self—for example, just chilling out on the sofa with our nearest and dearest or relaxing when out to dinner with a close friend—has now become prime opportunity for social media updating, tagging and posting that requires the continuation of this pressure to perform. We are never far away from the need to present a false-self, thus creating an entire generation, possibly an entire world, of people who don't know how it feels to be at peace with who they are, who don't know what it's like to spend time away from the pressure to be seen as perfect and acceptable, which, as a side effect, is quite possibly leading us to a world full of sadness.

So, now it's time to start to turn the spotlight around onto you personally as we begin to take some time for you to recall your own experiences when you felt the need to project a false-self.

Let us start to open this up by journaling the answers to the following questions. Just jot down the first response that pops into your head.

What parts of myself do I know that I most commonly hold back or cover up?

What do I present instead? Can you describe how your false-self shows up?

What are the most common situations that lead me to feel I need to cover these parts of me up?

What scares me most about showing up as my true-self?

Showing up to these places as our true-self will naturally create a level of anxiety. We have to accept that we are putting ourselves out there for all to see, and there will always be an element of risk with that. Brené Brown, PhD, a shame and vulnerability researcher, helps us to further understand that this is a vital part of the process. Through her work, she explains that these feelings of worry and anxiety that flood through us in response to facing this fear head-on are also vital key-holders to our ability to experience feelings of joy, aliveness, creativity and individuality.

If we don't allow our true-selves to be seen and embraced, instead choosing to continue to project a false-self, we also give up the chance to feel genuine joy and experience true acceptance. By not showing the world our true self, yes, we may feel protected from the hurt that we feel from the possible rejection we fear, but we are also turning our back on some of the most fulfilling emotions, connections and feelings that we could know and fully experience.

When one is stuck in a rut of continually presenting a false-self, it makes it incredibly difficult to establish real, genuine connections with others. How can we truly feel that sense of deep, lasting connection when the 'us' we are trying to establish in such a connection is ultimately false?

Ever notice how you have specific people who you feel incredibly safe with? Those who you feel you can relax fully around and have a deep sense of connection with? Take a second and think about what image you project when you are around them. I would hasten a bet that you don't project *any* image and that these are actually the people who you can be around as your true-self, without fear of any judgment.

So, what makes you feel able to be your true-self around these people? Being totally comfortable as 'you' with them is likely because you feel worthy of their love, unconditionally, which leads to a real sense of belonging. *These* are the connections we need to nurture and cherish. When feeling the need to present a false-self, we are attempting to nurture the wrong connections. We will never find a true sense of peace around those for whom we feel the need to change who we are in order to be accepted. If we spend our days fiercely trying to fit in to the crowds that we think we should be fitting in to, projecting the person we think we *ought* to be, we are also neglecting the real, true connections that matter. For it is these connections that will enable us to relax into being our true-self more and more. The more we allow ourselves to show up as our true-self, the less we'll feel comfortable in the situations that demand we change.

I must make a point here about context, because—as with everything—context is king. Adjusting behavior for a social context is *not* the same as projecting a false-self. To act the same, with no filter, in every situation in your life is not the goal here. We always need to understand that context still counts in how we alter our behavior around others, but to be authentic while doing so is always possible. We can still be our true-self and at the same time tone down our language when we're in a job interview, choosing different words and mannerisms than we would use while out at a bar with a friend, for example. Just like we can show our true-self but be far more animated and playful when talking to our partner than when we are talking to our boss or the next-door neighbor. I think you get my drift.

So how do we know when we are projecting a false-self? Well, you will feel it. And the less and less you do it, the more obvious it will become when you do. Spending a day, or even a few hours, projecting an image that isn't really you can become exhausting and you will more than likely tire far more easily in these situations. If you are unsure, just take a moment to ask yourself whether you are acting and speaking in total harmony and compatibility with your true-self and core values? Are you second-guessing your words all the time or worrying about what others will say? Are you running scripts though your mind before you speak, preparing and practicing certain conversations? Are you having to change your thoughts or beliefs to fit into the conversations around you? Are you having to present mistruths as to how you really feel about something?

I used to get absolutely exhausted when I was called to attend fitness exhibitions and seminars, which was unfortunate because I used to go to a lot of them. The memories of having to go and walk around, projecting an image to comply with what I considered would be expected became a real issue for me. I'd be shattered for about a week afterwards. It was like a hangover, but from appearance-presenting instead of wine. Certainly not as fun! The more I became aware of myself doing this, the more I could see clear indicators of so many others doing exactly the same. I would look at people as we chatted and I would be looking into the eyes of someone who was completely shattered and deeply insecure about who they were, yet they'd be totally focused on projecting an image that was displaying the complete opposite.

When I decided to just be honest about this feeling of dread that I would get in anticipation of attending these events, I could have been fearful about how people would respond as a result. I was taking a risk by admitting it because, at the end of the day, I was still a coach and most would expect me to feel at home in the atmosphere at these shows and exhibitions. However, after openly discussing this, many other coaches contacted me and told me that they felt exactly the same way. Many other coaches were exhausted with all the falseness and the pressure to 'perform' at these places too, but the fear behind the shame of being seen for what was behind the disguise meant that they felt stuck and unable to do any different for fear of judgment and criticism from their peers.

Can you see how easy it becomes to end up in a situation where not one single person in a room is there as their true-self? Which means that, when we are choosing which image to present, we may be trying to mold ourselves to fit in with someone else's false-self, who in turn is trying to fit in with the next person's false-self—resulting in an entire room of false-selves! It happens in the fitness industry all the time and doesn't just affect the coaches, of course. It affects you, the clients, too. Gym classes, diet clubs, health clubs… there will always be people in those environments who feel unable to show their true-self for fear of what 'people will think,' but the only question we need to ask at this moment in time is, are you one of them?

The truth is, we cannot control how other people view us. Other people's opinions of us are, of course, totally subjective. One person's view of someone else can be radically different from someone else's view of the same person, so trying to exert any control over how we are viewed by anyone other than ourselves is pointless. We also need to remember that the outer image we project is often a reflection of the one thing that we are trying to cover up. You can tell a lot about a person's fears by assessing how they react to you. For example, if someone was to measure their own worthiness by how slim they are, then they will likely judge you on that same basis. If someone was to base their own worthiness on how much money they make, they'll judge you on that information, too. We judge the world by how we judge ourselves.

This is why people who are obsessive about specific diet protocols or training methods think that everyone *else* should be doing these things too. My way or the highway, so to speak. Social media is full of examples of this as people project their own ideals and views onto others as gospel, merging their own self-judgment out onto the rest of the world—if eating clean and never having bread is how they become 'good enough' in their own eyes, then they'll feel that's how you should be showing your worth, too.

When we settle into a life where we are more comfortable in presenting our true-selves as standard, we also learn to release ourselves from the judgment of others. If we no longer feel a need to judge ourselves, we no longer feel a need to judge other people. Releasing yourself from the shackles of judgment—on both sides—can be powerful. Can you imagine how liberating that would feel?

The act of judging others less, helping you to judge yourself less, will happen naturally as you do the focused work within yourself. There are three ways that we can start to be released from the judgments we place onto others right now. By implementing these at the beginning of the action process, getting to grips with this will then leave more room for us to work on ourselves.

Try to understand that you very rarely know everything about a person, so is it really acceptable for you to make a judgment about them? If you find yourself starting down a slippery path of judgment towards another person, STOP and ask, "Do I really know enough about them to make this judgment?"

Lean in and turn the focus back onto you. Ask "Where is this judgment coming from within me, and why has it hit such a nerve?"

Ponder how you could change this thought to bring to it a more positive and accepting focus.

## 24

# Who the Hell Are YOU?

So how do we do this then, how do we start to live without this need to project a false-self? How do we learn to embrace who we are without that all-consuming, constricting fear of judgment? Well, first, in order for you to show your true-self more, we need to find out who you actually are.

We need to go deep beneath all the shoulds, woulds, oughts and find out what makes you *you*.

Your true-self is you at the core of your being. It isn't the roles you play or the identities that you have adopted during your life. Your true-self isn't found by labeling yourself as a mother, a wife or a sister, it's not your profession, nor is it your adopted role as a caregiver for your family. Your true-self was you before all this came about, the person that exists behind all these labels that have been attached to you. Your true-self is the woman who would show up and slap you in the face should you ever be presented with your own imminent death. Your true-self is the woman who speaks in the silence between your 70,000+ thoughts in a day. It is the woman who whispers to you as you fall asleep about all of the lost dreams, goals and talents you've let fall away from your life.

So how can we begin to identify more with her? Well, first, let's look at the evidence of where she has shown up most in the past.

Usually we are taught to create a list of 'wants' to identify our ideal life, but once again, Brené Brown is on hand to help here as she suggests that, instead, we should be looking at the evidence of where the joy has *already* shown up and been evident in our lives. For we never really know that having more money, living in a different place or being a different size or shape will make us feel happier. We are assuming, guessing, so instead, let's start by creating a 'joy list.'

We are going to look back over your life and begin to identify when and where you experienced the most joy.

When have you felt most at peace?

At what times in your life have you felt worthy and 'enough' as you were, unconditionally?

When were the times that you recall experiencing the most unconditional joy, laughter and connection?

Describe what was happening around you. Where were you? Who was there? What was the environment like?

Create a list of the most joyful times you recall and write down every detail about what things made these times feel so good to you.

Now, hold those memories in your mind as we start to bring it back to the present.

What makes your current experiences different from these?

What is missing now that was evident in these joyful experiences?

By doing this task, you will begin to learn what circumstances enhance your ability to feel at ease, at peace with yourself and able to experience true joy. Rather than attempting to guess at what will create joy in the future, we now have some solid evidence of those feelings to work with.

# 25

# FEEL the Fear

In this day and age, we are used to doing absolutely everything that we can to avoid that feeling of taking a risk, as we are taught that vulnerability is a bad thing. We fear it more and more as we age, simply because we have spent so long learning how to avoid it. Everything I am asking you to do will take an element of courage. There will be a lot of 'firsts' as you do things that you have previously not let yourself do or avoided because you felt uncomfortable doing it. You will be making choices that you have previously avoided making, and that familiar feeling of butter-flies in your gut will become commonplace for a while as you dive into this process. Even so, as each 'first' passes by, you'll begin to experience the real sense of release that comes along with courage. It takes ultimate courage to be seen in all our rawness, but it also presents to us the ultimate freedom.

If we watch children, we can see how it works to show up as our authentic true-self without fear. It's only as we grow older that things start to change, as we are taught about the need to change who we are to conform to standards in order to 'protect' ourselves from the risk of judgment from others. Once we have had an experience where we are judged harshly for a part of us, we recognize that it hurts us and thus we learn to do what we can to ensure that we never feel that hurt again. It isn't long until nearly every aspect of us will have been judged at some point, therefore everything that was once authentic about us ends up hidden from public view.

As a child, it may have taken just one playground quip or a brief comment from another kid, or even from a teacher, to initiate this subconscious thought chain reaction. Then as adults, we get bombarded every single day with images and ideals about who we should and shouldn't be that are having the same effect as these words we heard as a child. If you are constantly presented with the message that being 'enough' and worthy is associated with being slim, toned and tanned, then every part of your body that you feel doesn't match up to that ideal gets hidden from view while you try to 'fix' it.

The anxiety you feel when ordering your food in a restaurant, then eating it in front of strangers or people you don't really know. That nagging feeling when you are working out, worrying that you are doing something wrong or that you don't look perfect enough while doing it. The constant checking in the mirror for the tiniest lump or bump before you head out for a night out. All of these habits have been created by thoughts that lead to a belief that leads to a behavior. Your true, authentic self would understand that what you order, or how you eat it, has nothing to do with your worthiness or 'enoughness.' Your true-self knows that you are worthy of love and belonging whether you choose to order and eat a salad *or* a double bacon cheeseburger. You are allowed to eat what you want! You are good enough to be here and you are good enough to be loved, no matter what.

Your everyday environment will have a huge effect on how easy you find this journey towards self-acceptance and authenticity. Having already spoken about certain situations that may exacerbate your fears of unworthiness, you may already have an inkling as to what needs to change in your life in order to move yourself away from these situations. It's important that you are prepared to change aspects of your life in order to allow these changes within to happen, because if you repeatedly put yourself back into a situation that you know leaves you feeling small, inadequate or not 'enough' then you are going to keep those feelings alight within you.

You see this often with women and their friendship groups. Take a moment and think about a group of women whom you know or have known that you always feel or felt a little awkward around. They may have been friends or just distant acquaintances, but every interaction (even a brief one) with them left you feeling anxious, inadequate and a bit down on yourself. Can you think of a group like this? Right now, this is a toxic environment for you to be in because of the way it makes you feel. There could be two reasons for this: the first is that you have been trying to mold yourself into a group of people who are presenting false-selves, making achieving any solid and authentic connections very unlikely. Or it could be that your fear of their judgment is making *you* show up to the situation projecting something other than your true-self in order to fit in with them, once again making it unlikely that the connections you make will be genuine. Either way, the solution is the same—removing yourself from the environment until you have done the work on yourself. Once you are comfortable disposing of your false-self protection mask and spending more time in your life as your true-self, you can then make a call as to whether you choose to re-integrate with this group or not. By then, you may have decided that it's not worth risking a return to the negative feelings and you may automatically find yourself mixing with a more authentic group of friends.

Remember, embracing that risk of showing up to a situation as *you* has the potential to create life-changing friendships and relationships. There will be times you still feel fear and you want to project something else but, honestly, what is the worst that could happen? You could get rejected. In fact, we all will face rejection of varying degrees and sorts for our entire lives. Whether it's the real you or the false one, there will always be people out there ready to try and tear you down. But rejection gives you the chance to move on swiftly, because those who don't embrace you are not the sort of connections that will serve you anyway. Recognizing this gives you power. If you were to respond to the rejection by trying to morph yourself into someone they *will* accept, they will never ever know the true you, resulting in a connection based upon fabrication. Save your time and energy, as it could be spent fostering and harboring the bonds that will enhance your life and leave you feeling a sense of real joy and belonging.

# 26

# Self-Limiting Beliefs

Limiting beliefs that we hold about ourselves and the world around us can lead to limiting behaviors in response. To get to know your true-self, it is important that first you are able to identify which of these self-limiting beliefs are contributing to your lack of self-worth, the feelings of not being good enough as you are.

Throughout the course of your life, mostly when you were growing up, you sucked in information into your subconscious mind just like a sponge sucks up water. You picked up snippets of conversations, comments, media stories, family values and teachings from your family, peers and the people around you, ultimately creating the world you see from within your mind today.

As we grow, our subconscious minds grow with us. This part of the mind is in charge of over 90% of our daily actions and thought patterns. It controls the beliefs about the world that we hold and the stories that we tell ourselves. Your subconscious mind is vastly powerful!

It comes as no surprise when you see the way the media influences us today that so many of us have subconscious beliefs that tell us that we are not quite acceptable as we are.

A passing comment about your new dress that you took the wrong way, a magazine article about a new diet that created a feeling of guilt or shame about your body shape, a lifetime of hearing people judge you and others on their weight—these have all been stored up, repeatedly strengthened over the years and harbored for so long that you now believe that is a hard fact that you are not good enough as you are.

Whatever you think about most, your subconscious mind will

strengthen, just like paths in a field. The well-worn and trodden-down paths are the easiest and most likely paths to take; the most common thought patterns that you have in your mind become the easiest ones to repeat. Many of these will be the exact same thoughts you had yesterday, and the day before, and the day before that.

These thoughts and beliefs that exist within your subconscious mind ultimately determine how you live, what you think, what you believe you can and can't do, what decisions to make and what you hold true about the world around you. Your subconscious mind likes to be proven right so it will readily search outwardly for confirmation of what you already believe to be true. Hence, we often seem to be attracted to the same type of experience, people and feelings repeatedly over the course of our lives. You are subconsciously seeking out affirmations which conform to the beliefs you already hold. Your subconscious acts like your own internal Sat Nav; its job is to keep you on the path that it already knows. In other words, it's directing you continuously back into your comfort zone. Whether or not that comfort zone is useful, true or beneficial to you, it doesn't care. It's just believing what you have taught it to believe, like a mirror reflecting back to you the thoughts you have fed it. Your subconscious cannot distinguish between what is real and what isn't.

Of course, this can create massive problems when your subconscious beliefs are all to do with how you are not worthy enough, not slim enough or not pretty enough. Because of how your subconscious mind works, if you were to try and show up for the rest of your life as your true-self, without first doing the exercises in Part Three, you might find it difficult because you would be going up against your own subconscious beliefs that tell you that the protection of a false-self is needed to be accepted. Your subconscious will continue to run the scripts that have convinced you that you are not good enough, thus making it hard for you to really enjoy the process of releasing your true self to the world.

This is why I have included the upcoming in-depth practical section. It's important for you to understand not only *why* you feel so down on yourself all the time, but how to change this and what you need to do in order to change these subconscious thoughts that are holding you back.

For any thought to become a belief, we first of all have to accept it as true—if you do not accept a thought as true, it will not become a belief. So, in order to feel confident, empowered and self-assured in your own unconditional worthiness, we first have to track back to where your thoughts of *un*worthiness began in order to find out what triggered those beliefs, and then we have to challenge them, break them down and create some new ones.

There are many reasons that we stay stuck in the repeating scripts of our self-limiting beliefs. Let's look at the four Es of self-limitation:

**Experience**—We act when something happens and we then draw conclusions, then inadvertently seek out the same outcome next time to confirm our beliefs, keeping us in our comfort zones and 'safe.'

*We learn our belief systems as very little children, and then we move through life creating experiences to match our beliefs. Look back in your own life and notice how often you have gone through the same experience.*
—Louise L. Hay

If your subconscious has stored the belief that you need to be of a certain weight or size before you feel confident, your subconscious will continually try to get confirmation of this belief. Meaning it's likely that you'll associate any feelings of dented confidence as automatically to do with your weight—even if in reality, there was no connection at all.

**Education**—We can't rely on direct experience for everything, so we learn the rest from the world around us. We listen to our friends' views on what is and isn't possible, to what our teachers tell us we can and can't do. We take these views as fact. In similar fashion, if we listen to our mother talk constantly about weight and how she wants to be thinner, and we hear our friends talking about the latest diet that the celebs who look so pretty are following, we are subconsciously being shamed about our body size before we even know what a diet is.

The shame we feel when exposed to this information at a young age will get stored into our subconscious and it'll create a stubborn (and fact-based, as far as you believe) viewpoint that, in order to be liked, pretty and accepted, you have to be thinner.

**Errors of logic**—We generalize everything. We go off hunches based more on subconscious fears than on the reality of the situation before us. The word 'because' can become extremely harmful as it gives impressions of us using a good reason, when that may not actually be the case. "I need to be slimmer to feel good about myself because..." This isn't a fact, it's a belief. A belief that being slimmer will give you something that you haven't got. This belief, as we've already established, isn't based on fact, but because you place the word 'because' in there, it takes on the guise of fact.

**Excuses**—We often feel the need to excuse ourselves from what we believe to be our limitations and likely failures. When we do something that doesn't work, we tend to want to leave ourselves blameless, so we use our limiting beliefs as a justification as to why it didn't work. "I didn't get the job because I'm too big, not attractive enough or too dumb for it." These again are all beliefs—not facts. The *fact* was likely that you just had the wrong experience or qualification for what the interviewer was looking for.

"See, I told you I couldn't do it!" How many times have you secretly had some element of pleasure when you have proved yourself right about something you couldn't do? I know I can recall many times when I experienced this as a child. This is your subconscious trying to validate those limiting beliefs.

These limiting beliefs are very often, once again, fear-based: we fear that if we go against the beliefs, somehow we will be harmed. If we stride out of our comfort zone and tackle obstacles in a different way, we fear ridicule, criticism or rejection by others as a result and this fear is enough to powerfully inhibit us. Our self-limiting beliefs can continue to back us even further into a corner. Believing the scripts and blaming what we have programmed ourselves to believe means that we do not learn from our own mistakes, continuing to limit us further and further.

*Did you choose your identity consciously, or is it the sum total of what other people have told you, significant events in your life, and other factors that occurred without your awareness or approval? If you were to begin to define yourself differently, in a way that's more empowering and accurate for who you are today, how would you describe who you've become?*
—Tony Robbins

The power of your subconscious mind will be a key player in this process of self-belief and confidence-building. Getting to grips with this will also help you to get to understand the reasons that all of your previous diets and appearance-fixing behaviors haven't worked for you.

*Even though this book is about achieving a sense of unconditional worthiness, if you are reading this and you genuinely do have a need to lose weight for health reasons, then the work we do on the subconscious will also be the key to achieving this healthy weight maintenance long-term. It is an important part of everything we do, whether we want to release ourselves from emotional eating habits or let go of any unnec-essary restrictions or fears of food.*

As I talked about in Part One, the entire diet industry is based around the premise that we all have a bottomless pit of willpower that should suffice for us to achieve anything we wish. This disregards the complex relationship between the conscious self and the subconscious self. To not prioritize the reprogramming of the subconscious mind in behavior change is akin to ignoring the engine mechanics when manufacturing a car.

Take a second to recall: remember that your subconscious mind makes up more than 90% of your daily decisions, making it extremely difficult to create long-lasting behavior change without focusing on the subconscious beliefs that led to that behavior in the first place.

This works for both scenarios covered in this book, those who overeat or those who undereat. There is just as much power in the messages received from your subconscious mind to *restrict* certain food as there is to eat more of it.

When your conscious and subconscious mind are in conflict, your subconscious will always win. What we want is for your subconscious to be on your side, to work for you rather than against you, for it to work with your conscious mind as a partnership. We want your subconscious beliefs to be in unison with what you want in your life and to work with you, rather than against you, for what you want to achieve in the future.

The great thing about all this is that self-limiting beliefs can be changed. Whether it is a belief that you hold on to about having to be able to fit into a size 10 dress in order to feel good or a belief that eating a piece of cake makes you feel comforted, they can be changed to help you to lead an altogether far more peaceful and fulfilled life.

Your obsession with diets could quite easily have been passed down to you from your mother, grandma or even just your best friend at school. It may have escalated so much that now every time you read a magazine, see the fitspiration images or get caught up in talking about a new diet, the belief you hold about having to diet to feel worthy gets reinforced. This is all a part of the long trail of faulty belief patterns that have convinced you otherwise.

Before we move on, I want to answer something I get asked quite a lot. And that is "Why is it that we have such an easy time recalling the negative messages that confirm our limiting beliefs, and such a tough time recalling the positive ones that challenge them?"

Well, this is an interesting one. We have something in our brains called a 'negativity bias.' Simply put, our brains become more aroused and react more strongly in response to negative stimuli than positive. Unfortunately, this is automatic and starts to occur as soon as our brains begin to process information at a young age.

As the neuropsychologist Rick Hanson, PhD, puts it:

>...the brain is like *Velcro for negative experiences but Teflon for positive ones*...learning from your childhood and adulthood—both what you experienced yourself and saw others experiencing around you—is locked and loaded in your head today, ready for immediate activation, whether by a frown across a dinner table or by TV images of a car-bombing 10,000 miles away.

Right now it may feel as though we are all doomed to a life of unworthiness and that change is simply too hard with all this negative reinforcement around us. It may feel at times like our brains are trying to make it as tricky as possible for us, but remember—it *is* possible to make significant changes to how you feel about yourself. That is the most important aspect in my eyes—the initial acknowledgment that this change is possible—and coming to understand the extraordinary power that your subconscious mind has over your entire life. Once you have recognized that, the world really does become your oyster.

It is correct, though, that the work that it takes to create this change isn't easy. That is why you will become one of the minority who are able to focus on the enjoyment of their lives without this constant chatter of self-sabotaging thought. You'll be one of the few who can show up as your true-self to any situation and put yourself out there without the nauseating anxiety about what you feel you lack, leaving you open to deeper feelings of love, joy and connection. You will be able to live fully without having to exhaust yourself pretending to be someone different, no longer plowing through life addicted to changing who you are, but instead *embracing* who you are.

Up until now, it'll have been easier to listen to the negative messages that surround you. It's easier to do so simply because there are more of them and everyone else listens to them too. It's considered the norm to try and fight for your right of worthiness by chasing change. Whether it's by eating this way, training this way, looking this way or becoming that way, you end up constantly chasing after this carrot of perfection on the stick of physical change, when really, that carrot is not designed to be caught.

The practical steps covered in Part Three will be focused on changing how you think, changing how you act and thereby changing how you feel. However, it's not all going to be about changing your mindset, because I also want to help you to make some practical lifestyle changes within your external environment that will enhance these internal changes. First, I want to make an important point to highlight that the next section is all about the *doing*. You can read this book ten times over if you wish, you may feel better just knowing the truth behind what you've already read, you may feel that just understanding the hows and whys behind you getting caught up in the yo-yo diet world will help you to feel better in itself, but to truly see a change in how you feel, forever, the work in the following section will need to be done not just as a one-off, but on an ongoing basis. As I mentioned before, it's not easy. If it was, everyone would be doing it! You, however, are not everyone— you are you, and you are here for a reason. Whether you decide to work through all the sections at once or focus on one at a time is entirely up to you. Many find that they feel it's best to focus on one or two tasks at a time to ensure it doesn't become overwhelming, but, please, do what feels best for you.

I just want to add in a small section here on selfishness, as I know from experience that there will be some of you sitting there reading this and wondering if all this 'self' work is going to mean you have to become selfish. In fact, that's one of the most common questions I get asked: "Doing all this stuff for me and making myself the focus of my life, am I not being selfish?"

It's a funny thing, selfishness. Once again, this is something we have learnt to fear and avoid as a trait that makes us a 'bad' person. How often did you hear from parents, teachers and elders as you grew up that you "shouldn't be selfish"? However, when we were a child, not being selfish was highlighted in making points about sharing toys and packets of crisps, not putting our entire life on hold to prioritize other people's lives.

When I was growing up, I felt this innate fear of being seen as selfish. It was one of the many worries that plagued me. I would consistently give more time to other people than I was really comfortable with—not because I genuinely *wanted* to, but because I feared not doing so would make me *look* selfish. It was only after I'd started to do all of this work on myself that I realized just how much this fear affected parts of my business and my relationships. Why was I so anxious about this? Yup, you guessed—a fear of judgment. I had gotten used to projecting a self that was totally selfless, always putting other people first and basing all of my decisions on what suited everyone else, ignoring what I wanted or needed. This did nothing to serve me in the long run and fueled a growing sense of resentment within me. I know that I've lost countless hours of time doing things for others that were done out of feelings of having to rather than because I wanted to. Now, this isn't to say that doing things for others is a negative thing. Of course not. It's what makes the human race so special—that we are prepared to put ourselves out to help our friends, family or even strangers when they need us. Still, this is another great example of where context is always needed. What I started to understand was that it was okay to see myself as just as important as everyone else. I realized that being completely selfish or totally selfless are the black and white ends of the scale in this case and, as we've already discussed, I do tend to like things to sit in the vast gray area in-between, this being no different. Of course, it's essential to recognize that to be an effective parent, your child's needs often have to be prioritized over yours, or that to maintain a healthy marriage, you need to be aware of your partner's needs as much as your own, and it is lovely to be able to be there at the drop of a hat for those who need you. Even so, taking this selflessness to extremes is where the problems can start to arise. When trying to avoid this judgment of being selfish, we often end up completely ignoring our own needs as a reaction. We try to overcompensate for this fear within us by wanting to be seen to be living entirely for other people. Doing this out of fear as opposed to love means that we are the ones who end up suffering the fallout from the feelings of bitterness and exhaustion that come with it. Not only does this not serve *you* in the long run, it won't serve anyone else around you either. You can offer your family and friends so much more if and when you are functioning at your best. For example, we are all accustomed to the instructions we hear before taking off in a plane that include "Make sure to put your oxygen mask on first, and then assist children or other family members." To have a fully functioning, relaxed, happy you half of the time will serve them far better than having a frazzled, begrudging, stressed-out you the whole time.

You have to be able to know yourself well enough to understand whether something is important enough to put before your own needs or if you are simply doing it because you feel you have no choice. Remember—there is always a choice. You just have to have the confidence in making it.

One of the strange things about selfishness is that it only appears to make sense in one way. The next time someone asks (or demands) that you change *your* plans to do something for them, I invite you to flip this request over on its head. Instead of questioning your own selfishness and how you should put them first, why not question theirs? They are asking you to put their needs before your own. Hmm, is that selfish of them? Each time, just take a second to quietly ask yourself, *Are they being selfish asking this of me, knowing that I already had plans for myself?*

There will be times when you know that they aren't asking with any selfish intent, whether it be from sheer desperation or from simply not understanding fully the impact that their request will have on you. Your true-self will find these situations easier to deal with, because once you take the fear away, you will feel far more able to have a full and frank conversation about it in order to get this information rather than immediately saying yes and then begrudging it for the entire day, when it may not have even been that important.

It is hugely important to recognize that your own confidence and well-being will and does have a direct effect on everyone else around you. To plod through life disgruntled and resentful from consistently prioritizing the demands of other people will not have a positive effect on you or those you share your life with. Your true-self wants to be seen, valued and appreciated. Your true-self is positive, upbeat and light. To take your own well-being seriously is a sign of wisdom. Think about the oxygen mask instructions on a plane—you can't take care of another person's life if you aren't first looking after yours.

We have come to the end of this section and hopefully it has taught you more about where you are, why you are here and where this version of you came from. It is now time to say goodbye once and for all to the stories that you tell of why you aren't enough, about what you lack or who you feel you should be instead. From this day forth, I invite you to speak only of how deeply you love, how loud you laugh and of how great you truly are. The chapters containing your fears, anxieties and the conditions that you've previously attached to your worth are about to be closed, for you cannot turn the page on this new chapter until you are ready to let go of the old one. You have the ultimate control over how the next chapter pans out.

There is a reason that self-love, self-respect and self-worth by definition require a healthy 'self' and self-identity. You will never find them anywhere else. All of the power lies within you, so let's go and find it.

*Owning our story and loving ourselves through that process is the bravest thing that we will ever do.*
—Brené Brown

# Part Three

# 27

# Self-Worth

I recently conducted a private online survey about self-love, worthiness and confidence. I asked people I'd never had contact with or ever spoken with to complete it, and I got a lot of responses. I'm an emotional type and I don't mind admitting that. Yes, I cry at Christmas films and often feel a lump at airport arrival halls. So it may come as no surprise that, as I was reading through these survey responses, I did indeed shed a tear or two. It was pretty hard not to. Never before have I read such rawness from people I've never met or spoken to. Some were brutal. Brutal in the way that the loathing that was emanating from the words about how some women view themselves was just crushing to read. Even so, it served me, because what I was looking for was confirmation. I know that may sound harsh, but I wanted to check once again that women felt as bad about themselves as I thought. They do. No matter how many times I ask, and in what way, I always get the same responses:

"I will never be enough."

"I have no confidence in myself at all and probably never will."

"I can't accept myself—I don't even want to when I look like this!"

"I'm just not good enough to like who I am."

Don't get me wrong, there were a handful of encouragingly positive ones too. What surprised me the most was just how many answered 'no' when asked if they'd be interested in attending an event or having coaching in order to help them to make changes in how they felt about themselves. Some of the most harsh and self-deprecating answers came from those who then said they weren't interested in change. It got me wondering whether this is because feeling this way is seen as something that is just simply unchangeable.

As we've dissected previously, we spend so much time, money and effort on trying to fix the symptoms of the lack of confidence and self-esteem, whether it be through dieting, training, supplements, clothes, cosmetics or surgery. Once again, it confirmed to me that if these things worked, long-term, the survey would have outlined an entirely different picture. We'd have a nation of strong, confident, empowered women who consistently own the space they are in, who show up as they are and just *know* that they are worthy, acceptable and enough. They would hold none of the misconceived notions of "when I have lost this weight" or "when I get this job" or "when my friends are being good to me." *True self-worth needs no 'whens' attached — it is unconditional.* Still, more and more women are fighting more and more battles with who they are, engaging in daily mental arguments with themselves about how they need to be this, that or the other before they can be happy within themselves, chasing the impossible possibility of perfection.

There will always be someone out there waiting to knock you down. If we only seek to find our self-worth in the label of a smaller dress size, in the winning of a race or in the achievement of promotion, then we are handing over the reins of our self-worth to someone or something else's control. Our self-worth is so precious we should never, ever let that control fall from our own grasp. After all, what happens when those environments aren't there anymore? What happens if we were to get ill and couldn't train, what happens if we were to lose our job, what happens if our likes and dislikes change, what happens if life throws us a curve-ball that affects these conditions and takes the control away from us? Do we just give up, flop down and resign ourselves to being worthless? We certainly do not! The issue is that you can't just change how you feel with the click of a finger when you want to. Unconditional self-worth takes work to uncover, it takes effort and it takes *time* to reprogram your mind into believing that you are enough with or without these conditions.

Self-love means letting yourself shine through the rain, snow, thunder or brilliant sun. It means being able to show up to any situation and just know in your heart that you are worthy of feeling accepted, that you are good enough to take up that space and that you are confident in your ability to love and be loved. Self-love isn't a wishy-washy way of saying you can't have goals or take care of yourself. That would go against self-love. When you truly love someone, you want to take care of them; you want them to be healthy, to be strong and fit! What it also means is that if, one day, you wake up and think *You know what? I think I'd like to take an art class today instead of hitting the gym*, it means that your self-worth doesn't even flicker. You stay the same person even as you let your personal tastes and hobbies change. Self-love means that once you start to get older and you see your body start to naturally change—a few inches here and there, a change in shape—you can view this with grace and without any paralyzing fear that you are going to have to spend the last twenty years of your life feeling worthless just because your body changed.

Self-love means you stay *you* and you stay confident, accepting and compassionate towards yourself, no matter what external, out-of-your-control conditions are presented to you. You can lead your life in ways that make you happy without fear that it will result in you losing your worth as a woman. And *that* is the purpose of what we are about to embark on. The practical tasks ahead were all at one time part of my own journey of change, and now they signify the beginning of *your* journey of change. So, if you are ready, and I think by this point you are, let's delve into action.

## 28

# Body Image

When it comes to improving the way we view our body, most people tend to think about changing it and altering how they look, but in fact it is building self-esteem that will make the most difference, not 'fixing' our self-image.

Concerns with weight often come from those who already have a negative body image. There is an obvious string of connections between hating how you look and having an obsession with dieting and appearance-fixing behaviors. However, the connection is maybe not as simple as you'd expect, because having a negative view of oneself does not automatically come as a result of your physical attributes, but from how you *feel* about them. So the body you live in doesn't determine your self-worth and self-esteem; the way you *feel* about the body you live in does, and as you know now, the way you feel can be changed, thus meaning your body image perceptions can be changed too.

Having a positive body image encompasses many elements. To name a few:

- Accepting your body as it is, enjoying it and having a realistic perception of it
- Acknowledging and understanding that bodies come in all shapes and sizes, and that no one shape or size is better or worse than others
- Knowing that our sense of character, and our worthiness as a person, is separate from how we look
- Accepting that physical appearance says little about the person underneath it.

All these points will have the benefit of ensuring that a person will likely naturally avoid becoming over-consumed with dieting, exercise, calories or weight. So it makes sense to understand that the majority of those who become stuck in a persistent long-term yo-yo diet cycle have a negative body image. This will likely see the opposite feelings and behaviors to those above, leaving us with a tendency to become far more obsessed with food, diets or exercise regimens.

There is also a strong connection between having a poor body image and falling prey to other related conditions such as stress, anxiety, sexual dysfunction, depression and, of course, eating disorders.

To give examples of a few characteristics of negative body image:

- Experiencing feelings of shame, anxiety or feeling awkward about your body
- Feeling that body shape, size or looks are an important factor in self-worth
- Having a distorted perception of body shape and/or size.

I would suggest that if you are reading this book, you may well recognize yourself to a certain extent within the above list. Although I hope that by this point, you'll also have recognized some movement towards the positive body image list also. Certainly you will by the time you reach the end.

Much of your own body image will have been decided as you were growing up because this still lies in your subconscious mind. As we move through this last section, the practical tasks presented will all play a role in changing the way that you see yourself. Pretty much everything we do from this point on will play a role in reprogramming your subconscious mind to lead with new, positive thoughts, feelings and beliefs, meaning that the way you see yourself will change, how you live your life will change and the self-limiting beliefs that have been holding you back will change.

So let's start with looking at how you view your body and what we can do to help shift these thoughts into self-love mode.

Unless you are a model or physique competitor, my first piece of advice would be to dump the before-and-after photos as a method of external validation of any fitness-based 'success.' We have seen why photos alone are a dangerous method of assessment and it's obvious that a headless bikini shot tells us nothing about fitness levels, happiness or psychological health. So if you are keen to keep a record of a fitness or dieting-based journey for health (and from a logical perspective, not emotional), then at least let's start to move away from this trend of abs-tell-me-all and incorporate different methods of judgment, some that will actually mean something to you, while also helping to improve your body image long-term.

Here are some ideas of what you can start to use as your own methods of assessment in these areas:

- Strength progressions
- Movement progressions
- Fitness progressions
- Mindset shifts
- Psychological health
- Overall happiness
- Body image
- Confidence
- Relationship with food

You can assess every single one of these without the need for a before-and-after shot.

*If you find that your coach still insists on getting a before-and-after shot from you, think wisely about their reasons for doing so. If it's not needed for your validation of your successes or worth, then it shouldn't be required for them either — unless they are more interested in their own promotion, which should be taken as a warning signal.*

# 29

# Finding Your Why

I want to talk more on motivation, because this fits in very well with the points I have just been talking about. The majority of the defense behind these before-and-after shots stems from the fact that most people who value these photos have entered into their fitness or diet journey from a 'looks' perspective, as opposed to overall enjoyment or long-term health, so see these photos as a viable method of judging overall success, meaning that their 'why' for working out and dieting is based on the 'looking better' mode of motivation.

Before we move on, I want you to start to make a list of all the reasons that you work out and diet. List as many as you can. Pretend you are answering the question spontaneously and naturally, without a lot of worry about what your answers sound like or if they are the 'right' ones.

Once you have done this, look through your answers and answer these two questions:

How many of my reasons are to do with the perceived 'reward' of what I will get as a result of working out or dieting? (For example, having a different body, winning a competition etc.)

How many of my reasons are to do with the enjoyment of these behaviors, actually liking the day-to-day 'doing' of dieting and working out? (For example, really enjoying the act of working out and choosing the diet-based food choices from taste rather than perceived reward)

As I mentioned briefly earlier in the book, it is helpful and important to honestly review and assess your motivations. This is important because it will affect not only your results, but it also plays a role in your body image. The first question that I asked, about the perceived reward, would show us how extrinsically motivated you are, whereas the second question will have highlighted how many intrinsically motivational factors are involved.

*Remember, extrinsic motivation is motivation that comes from an outside source, where you are motivated based on a highly regarded outcome or ego-boosting reasons, rather than the enjoyment of the activity itself. Intrinsic motivation is motivation from within, stemming from the enjoyment of an activity or skill solely from the satisfaction of enjoyment, learning or having fun.*

So what does all this have to do with body image? Well, it has been shown in studies that a keen interest in health, fitness and nutrition from *intrinsic* motivation plays a role in fostering body-image satisfaction. Whereas entering into the world of fitness or dieting purely from an extrinsic motivational standpoint—shame- or guilt-based need to appearance-fix—can lead to poorer psychological well-being, as well as lower self-esteem and overall health, all of which have a negative effect on our overall body image.

*Plus extrinsic-based motivation can also lead to a tendency for shorter-term adherence (hence the yo-yo element)—*Maltby & Day, *Personal Motivation, Body Image, Health Behavior and Stage of Exercising.*

It becomes important therefore to ensure that your motivations for exercise and/or eating well have an element of intrinsic motivation at their roots. The simplest way of doing this is to prioritize the activities that you enjoy. If you embark on a training regime purely because you have heard that it's good for weight loss, but you don't really enjoy it, then how long do you think you'll keep that behavior up? Any activity that sees you moving regularly for the next ten years is far more effective than an activity that sees you moving more, but only for six months. The same logic applies to food: when following a diet where you only have a few sources of allowable foods or where you've been told that steak for breakfast is the only option (even if it makes you gag), how long do you think it will last? The easiest, most effective and certainly the most common-sense approach would be to seek out the activities that you actually enjoy doing and eat the foods that you can appreciate and savor. You can still eat well and enjoy it. The two aren't mutually exclusive, no matter what you may have been told.

We are coming to the end of this first section, so let's recap the tasks above that you can start to do today to start this process of change:

Assess your level of motivation for every activity you are currently doing. Is your reason for taking part purely extrinsic? If so, what can you do to bring more intrinsic motivation into these activities?

What other activities could you start to do more of that you know you would truly enjoy?

What needs to change in order to make your current habits more enjoyable?

Change your methods of assessment in your health and fitness-related goals so that your progress becomes focused on what you do and how you feel, rather than how you look. Get used to determining your success on these factors by watching how you speak about your journey. For example, if someone asks you how your training is going, then respond by making a point about how much stronger you are or how much you are enjoying it. If someone asks you about your food choices, then answer by explaining how good it makes you feel and how much you enjoy eating it. If you find you are having to lie (and wear your disguise of enjoyment) about these things, then that is a good indication to go back and reassess your motivations once more.

## 30

# Your Values Are Your Future

*Happiness is not something ready-made. It comes from your own actions.*
—Dalai Lama XIV

So, what are values? Values compound the things in life that are important to us, the things that matter to us, what we hold dear to us and that make us who we are as people. The things that make us individuals. To live a life aligned to your own core values is to pave your way to living your own truth and happiness.

Society has no right to dictate to you what you want from your own life, nor have your parents, friends or teachers. It's highly important here that you start to recognize what idea of society you may have adopted as your own and where your own ideal lies in comparison to this. Only then will you be able to suss out if you are actually living your life in accordance with the life you truly want to live or if you have just fallen prey to living the way you think you *should* be living.

This task is about finding your own five core values and then ensuring that you can see evidence of these within your own life. You will value different things from the next person—no two people will have the same list. If you take some time to understand the real priorities in your life, what you truly love and what makes you happy, then you'll be able to determine the best direction for you as you move on into the future. Figuring out your own life values will help you make decisions like:

What job should I pursue?
What hobbies should I prioritize?

Should I accept this promotion?
Should I start my own business?
Should I compromise or be firm with my position?
Should I follow tradition or travel down a new path?
Should I buy that new house or car?

When the actions you take, the way you live and your behaviors all match your values, life tends to be good—you feel satisfied and content. But when your day-to-day life doesn't align with your personal values, that's when things feel, well, a bit wrong. This can end up being a real source of unhappiness and disconnection for many.

It is easy to get caught up in a trap of thinking you have to do what is expected of you, but this is just another self-limiting belief. Ultimately, you are in control and it's you who will be living the consequences of any decisions you make for the rest of your time on this planet. So it's vital to ensure that the future consequences of any decisions you make fit in well with what *you* want from life.

Once you start to break down the list of your values to a shortlist of your core five, you will be able to find examples of each that are already a part of your everyday life. However, that said, it may also feel obvious that there is a huge lack of evidence for holding these values. If this is you, no need to worry—worry is banned—you can view this as a positive thing as you have plenty of opportunity to start to find ways in which you can increase the evidence of these five things in your life, which even in itself will have a huge impact on your day-to-day feelings about life.

Your core values will also help you to understand the burning questions of "Who am I?" and "What do I stand for?" which will fit in very well with the rest of the work we do. When you think about these two questions as you read them now, you may get worried as you realize that you have no idea of the answers. You may even have been used to making something up to fit with whatever disguise you were wearing at the time, but that's okay. The amount of people I work with who have no idea what their *values* are is to me a strong clue that they also have no real idea who *they* are.

Alternatively, you may already have an inkling as to what your values are. However, I'd still recommend that you do the tasks again now, having gotten yourself into an open, ready-to-change mindset. There have been instances where I have introduced values with a client and it turns out that the values they presented to me originally were not their true values. They were the values that they *thought* they should have.

Why are values so important? Well, most of us fall into default mode in life far too easily. We leave school with no idea what we want to do, where we want to be or what we are even good at and, as a result, we fall into the trap of getting a job, *any* job. In our contemporary global economy, we have become even more fearful about this constant threat of 'lack' that the media presents to us over our breakfast every day. It has created a society where to have any job, even one we hate, is something we are to feel grateful for. Any life, even one we hate, we are to feel grateful for.

Because of this thought process being encouraged to us right from the ground up when we are children, it creates a society where people rarely have a clue about what they truly want out of their life. We have been conditioned to live in an 'accept' state of mind and, to some extent, we are encouraged to feel guilty for wanting something else for ourselves. We certainly aren't encouraged to delve deep within and find out our true passions and follow our dreams. It is seen as self-indulgent to want to be happier and to want to improve our day-to-day fulfillment, so instead we sit back and let life do its thing around us, the control well and truly left in the hands of other people.

People who pursue other things and push their lives to follow a different path are then seen as outliers, lucky or privileged. They are often held in contempt by others as they are viewed with suspicion and, truthfully, jealousy. However, these folk aren't outliers, they are just *people*, but people who decided they wanted more, who decided they wanted to make a difference, who wanted to follow a path in life that made them happy. They followed their own heart, no one else's. They knew exactly what they wanted and went for it with full confidence that they could make it happen. To understand your core values is an essential part of this process of change, because it will enable you to understand what is lacking in your current life that is important to you.

It is key to understand here that while we do strive for change, it is important to do so with a feeling of gratefulness for what we have now. This is absolutely essential for our well-being and living a happy and emotionally fulfilled life. A daily practice of expressing gratitude for what you have (while embracing future change) is important, so much so that I have included a small section on this later on. For now, though, we need to identify your values:

Start by journaling the answers to the following questions. Grab your pen and notepad and just start to write. Don't overthink these questions. Just go with what comes to you. Remember, this is all about getting past the disguise and identifying what makes the person behind it.

Identify the times you have felt happiest (use times from at work or personal life).

Identify the times you were most proud of your achievements (be truthful—think about the times you felt proud in yourself, rather than proud of the praise received by others).

When do you feel you're most fulfilled and satisfied?

When do you feel most at peace?

What memories and experiences make your heart smile?

Go back to when we talked about you being able to be your true-self. When are you able to take off all your masks and be yourself without fear?

What are the common denominators of the experiences? Where were you? What were you doing? Who were you with?

Turn to the 'values list' at the back of this book and begin to circle or highlight the ones that best represent the common feelings that you felt with these experiences above.

You may find that some naturally fit together, for example, effectiveness & efficiency, or joy & laughter. Circle them all to begin with, then start to narrow them down to your Top 10.

Then we need to compact it down again to your Top 5 core values. Ask yourself, "If I had to satisfy and align my life with only five, which would I choose?"

Then look over your list first thing the next morning and ask yourself again, "Do these five values represent me at my very core?" Do they represent what you would support? Do they make you feel positive and energized so they give you that truthful gut feel of "This is me"?

If not, don't worry! Go back and repeat the process until you are 100% happy with your five.

When you are happy with your five core values that represent you at your rawest, your unmasked self, incorporate each one into a statement. For example, if you had picked "make a difference" then make a statement to complete the meaning like "I seek to make a difference with my life," "I seek to make a difference in the world," or "I seek to make a difference to those around me."

Once you find your core values, most self-help resources will leave it at that, but there is little point in having a list of values but no real idea how to apply them. The next step is making the choice to live with integrity towards your values and to use them to help you make future decisions, letting them become your moral compass, so to speak.

So now we'll do a small journal task to identify where your starting point is. Look around and identify where you see evidence of these values in your life as it is. Journal the answers to these questions:

Where do I see evidence of my core values in my current day-to-day life?

What needs to happen in order for me to become more aligned with and living in accordance with my core values each day?

Do my values match my current priorities?

By knowing your values, you will know what is most important to you. This is a vital step in getting to know your true-self. It's essential to know who your true-self is before you can expect yourself to show up and live fully as her!

Living in accordance with your values will mean that you can use them as a checklist for prioritizing. If we use our core values to help us to choose paths, make decisions and prioritize our time, then it's likely that every decision we take and every move we make will be in accordance with our true-self, meaning we are constantly moving towards situations that our true-self requires and feels comfortable being in, hence, a lesser need to wear a disguise.

This is why it is so hugely important to identify your own values as opposed to running your life via everyone else's. You may have picked up notions of what constituted important values from your parents, peers or even from society, so it's absolutely essential that you choose your values for you. Tune into your gut and ask one last time, "Are these core values mine or someone else's?"

Once you are 100% sure that they are all yours, with no external influence, then you are good to go. We can set the next phase in motion!

NB: You can change your values as your life progresses. They don't have to be static. For example, you may come to the conclusion that one of your values isn't leading you towards your best self (and therefore, best life). You may go from someone who values wealth as top priority to someone who values peace more. The key is to ensure that your values are accurate for your true-self in any given period.

Future 'check-in' journal question: "Does my day-to-day life match a life whose owner has these core values?"

Another way to tell if you are on the right track is that the decisions made off the back of your values will see your true-self showing up. The path that your values will lead you down will be one of integrity in line with who you are, thus no longer needing a disguise to hide under.

You may make a decision based on your values that you soon recognize wasn't in line with your true-self. For example: you say 'yes' to a week away at a fitness camp because your values listed "fitness," but as you show up to the camp, you realize that you feel that familiar feeling of wanting to wear a disguise, to portray someone different. Maybe you feel the need to be someone who is more 'into' this sort of fitness than you really are, or you feel the need to embellish the truth about your diet or fitness habits in order to fit in with the rest of the camp attendees. Whatever way you look at it, your true-self is not comfortable in showing up to that situation.

This doesn't mean that health isn't a core value for you; you just need to narrow it down to what the word 'fitness' actually means to you. Maybe your 'best' and happiest life would see fitness as being something you do in private? Maybe even changing your exercise routine to something entirely different. You can still prioritize your health and fitness, but ensure you are honest with yourself when evaluating which situations will make you want to wear your disguise and honor your true-self by scrubbing these situations off the to-do list.

This situation is what we call misalignment. Something just didn't quite match up to your values and your true-self. All this means is that it needs a bit of clarifying, so the next time you can make a more informed decision. In the example mentioned above, you'd either adapt the value to be more specific or scrap it and dig deeper to assess whether this was even a true value in the first place. If the latter is the case, what needs to replace it?

Your values will play a big part in the development of your self-esteem and overall happiness. The more you can live in alignment with them, the more you'll start to live as your true-self, creating a happier, healthier and more fulfilled you.

# 31

# Challenging Your Limiting Beliefs

We covered what self-limiting beliefs are earlier on, so you are aware of what they are and how you got them. In this section, we will start to look at how we can detach from them and create some new, more helpful beliefs to replace them.

Let's first take a look at a few common ones that you may or may not recognize. I'll list the ones I have seen most often in my coaching practice:

"I'm worthless as I am."

"I can't love myself like this. I'm not good enough and don't deserve self-acceptance."

"If I don't constantly diet, I'll just let myself go and pile a heap of weight on."

"I have to train daily or I've failed myself."

"I screw up all the time. I can't seem to stick to anything."

"I've messed up now. I might as well just forget it and start again next week."

It's important to reiterate that these self-limiting beliefs are not fact. Each and every one of these common stated beliefs stem from your opinion. Because they have been repeated and relayed as fact over and over again within your mind for so long, they are now believed to be truth. Your subconscious feels the need to be right, and to do so, it will constantly search for evidence to back up these beliefs. So you may find that the situations that you find yourself in will often be perpetuating these beliefs within you. For example, spending time with others who believe those things, adding to your confirmation that they must be true. Hearing others relay their own beliefs as being the same or similar to yours will only compound that your beliefs are correct — this is why it's common for families to have very similar belief systems. It's going to be so important for you during this process to really look closely at how you spend your time and who with.

So, let's go back to those example beliefs. I'm going to list them again but, this time, I'm going to add some words in to make each of them a more accurate statement.

"I *feel* worthless as I am, because *I believe* that to be worthy, I have to look a certain way."

"I *feel* I shouldn't love myself like this. *I believe* that I'm not good enough and *feel* guilty and undeserving of self-acceptance."

"If I *choose* to not constantly diet, I *fear* that I will let myself go and pile a heap of weight on because I *don't trust* that I can control myself around food."

"I *feel* like I have to train daily or I *feel* like I've failed myself because my worth is judged on how I look."

"I make different *choices* to what I'd planned all the time. I *choose not* to stick to things because they are often unsustainable."

"I've *made a choice* that wasn't planned. I *choose* to enjoy it and let it go, for I understand that tomorrow is a new day."

Can you see the difference a few changes in the wording makes? These statements are now more accurate because we have established that the belief started within you and is based on opinion. Opinions that have been building up within you based on what your subconscious believes to be true, from all the messaging, conversations and images picked up along the course of your life. Remember, though, just because it's what you *feel*, it doesn't make it fact.

If you believe that your looks determine your worth, then they will. If you believe that you have to train every day in order to feel accepting of yourself, then you will need to.

The simple difference here is to change what you believe to be true. By changing what you believe, you will change how you feel, therefore rendering these statements redundant, giving yourself a chance to replace them with positive, self-accepting statements such as:

I always feel worthy, in every situation!

I'm in control of how acceptable I feel and I choose to feel full self-acceptance. I show the world how to treat me.

I am capable of health. I am capable of making positive decisions. I am capable of knowing what will serve me and my body and what won't.

I train because I want to train and enjoy it! I am capable of choosing when to work out and know that I am worthy with or without exercise every day.

I stick to what is sustainable for me. I embrace flexibility and trust myself fully and completely to make the decisions that are best for my true-self.

I choose to lead a lifestyle that I can adapt to my life, hobbies and preferences. Each day is unique and I trust myself to be able to handle it!

This seems quite a simple task when I do an example like this for you; however, we also have to accept that your current self-limiting beliefs have been stored within you, gaining more and more strength for a very long time.

So first, I want you to write down five of your most common self-limiting beliefs. Let's choose the ones that you feel keep you stuck in that yo-yo diet, weight-obsessed mindset. What self-limiting beliefs hold you captive to the diet industry? Which of your beliefs are the gurus hitting on when they sell you that dream of happiness via a smaller body?

Write them down one by one as you think them. They can be similar in wording. They just have to really mean something to you. If you read one and think, "Yeah, I never really think that," then scrub it out until you have a list of statements that you know and recognize to be your subconscious mind's favorite scripts.

Now we need to go back over each one and take out the definitive words that make it appear as fact. Look at where you have written "I am" or "It is" or "I can't" and so on. These sorts of statements often denote ideas we believe are facts versus opinions.

As such, it is helpful to change these to words that denote opinion instead, such as "I feel" or "I think."

Read through the statement again. How do you feel now that you can see that this statement is really just your opinion?

Now we need to compact down these statements into a list of solid conclusions and beliefs. Make a short list of the most common denominators, but still using the opinion words. For example:

My statements show that I believe…

"I feel I need to look a certain way in order to be acceptable."

"I don't feel I trust myself to be able to manage my own health and well-being."

"I believe I will only be happy when I look different."

"I don't feel good enough as I am."

The next part is figuring out where these beliefs originally came from so that we can challenge them even more. You know that you weren't born believing these things. When you were a small child, these statements would have seemed alien to you, but as you grew older and your subconscious started to take notes, they became ingrained statements that you have lived your life by ever since—deeply held beliefs that, in your mind, became 'facts'.

So get your journal again and make some more notes as we go. Start with the first belief, then slowly work through the questions for each one.

Think back over your life. When did this belief first start to show up for you?

Can you recall what was happening around you at that time of life? Who did you spend time with? Where did you go? What did you spend your time doing?

What sparked this belief in your mind? Where did this idea come from?

Who, or what, first introduced the belief to you?

Were they speaking from fact? Or were they just expressing their opinion on what they believed at the time to be true?

What was going on within them at that time that may have caused them to believe it?

Who may have taught it to them?

And, in turn, who may have taught it to them?

Is it absolutely, definitely, a fact?

Once you have completed these questions with all of your beliefs, you will be a little closer to finding the source of where they came from. The problem with self-limiting beliefs is, because they weren't based on fact in the first place, they have no boundaries. The beliefs quickly become like Chinese whispers, building up a powerful momentum that can result in you changing how you live your entire life, based on nothing more than what was originally a flippant comment. These beliefs do not work on logic. If you have believed that you need to be smaller to feel worthy, then you will always believe that you need to be smaller to feel worthy—even when you become smaller! That belief will not alter in response to external change. Meaning you will never escape that cycle of unworthiness that this belief has created within you.

These insecurities are not yours; they have merely been learnt. So don't claim them as part of your life story, since they don't belong to you. Now is the time to let those beliefs go and to recreate some new ones that will help you to move forward and live a life full of confidence and worthiness—because these beliefs are part of your new story. Are you ready to claim them?

# Self-Talk

Self-talk is another way of describing this internal dialogue we all have that is made up of different versions of those false beliefs we just discussed in the previous task. Now that you have begun to challenge the credibility of those beliefs about yourself that have been haunting your mind for so many years, they need to be replaced by new beliefs, ones that will instead help you to move forward in appreciation for who you are and what you do.

Imagine you are going back to when you were younger and your subconscious mind had only just started to take information in. Well, all we are doing is re-activating that process, but with more accurate and helpful information this time.

Earlier on, we determined your values. If when you were led to assess your current life for evidence of your core values, you struggled to find it, then this is a good indication that you have been living your life under the influence of self-limiting beliefs.

It is important that you create your new thoughts specific to those past negative beliefs that you picked out, so that each time your mind rattles off these old false beliefs, you have an immediate back-up answer to respond with. The subconscious mind works on repetition, so this will be a key aspect in having your subconscious accept these new beliefs as standard. Eventually, these new beliefs will begin to replay automatically like the negative ones used to. As you show up to the world as your true-self, take part in the activities that serve your best self and begin to live your life in an authentic and peaceful way, your subconscious will be right there with you helping to make it happen.

Take these statements one by one and first, out loud, acknowledge again that this statement is opinion, that it's based on someone else's insecurities and that you now choose to disown this belief as it no longer serves you.

Now we need to fire out some comebacks. I want you to say the belief in your mind while standing up and then physically move your position—walk to the other side of the room, turn around, just move—and then answer it back with an opposing statement. Use a positive affirmation that renders this old belief dead in the water.

Some examples using some slightly different limiting beliefs from earlier:

Original—"I'm not slim enough, so I need to try every diet I can find to fix it."
New—"I am strong. I am intelligent. I am healthy. I am enough. I am capable of taking care of myself and I trust my own body's wisdom."

Original—"I'm fat and ugly and people judge me because I'm not pretty or slim enough."
New—"I am worthy of love and acceptance, right now. I choose to surround myself with positive, kind people who I can be my true-self with and who love me unconditionally."

Original—"I'll never be able to change how I feel about myself!"
New—"The only person in control of how I feel about myself is me, and today, I choose to love and accept myself."

Once you have a list of your new, powerful statements, it now becomes about repetition—at the core of it, this is how the older, false beliefs became 'fact' in your head. You just replayed them over and over again, so now you do the same with the new ones.

A great time for your subconscious to be exposed to these new beliefs is when you are in a relaxed and open state. So I would recommend making a voice recording of all your statements and replaying them to yourself as you are lying down to sleep, and then once again in the morning as you wake.

If you feel icky about listening to your own voice, then get your partner or someone close to you to record them for you. This will also help as it's coming from another voice. You may find that you accept these statements from someone else more readily than you do yourself at this time. This is fine. You will begin to become much more open and trusting of yourself as time goes on.

I cannot stress how absolutely vital it is that this becomes an ongoing process. It's unlikely to make a difference if you only repeat these affirmations every few days or if you repeat them 25 times on the first day and then never again. The original false beliefs are still running on automatic, so you'll still be exposed to these until they are made completely redundant. The key is that every time you recognize an old self-limiting belief appearing in your mind, you react by affirming your new belief in response, out loud where possible. Thus, eventually, your new beliefs will become the automatic ones and finally you and your mind will both be fighting for the same thing—a happy, authentic and confident YOU!

## 33

# Setting Boundaries

As you begin to make the transition from fearful, conditional self-worth to confident, unconditional self-worth, you'll realize that it's going to take some initial long, hard looks at how you currently spend your time, who you spend it with and what information you readily accept into your mind each day.

Over the next two sections, we will be talking about setting boundaries, emotionally and physically, switching off from all the negative chatter around you that no longer serves you. By now, you should be knee-deep into the process of resetting your subconscious beliefs and that means that the old information sources that used to encourage your mindset of fear, lack and not-good-enough have got to go. If you feel unable to show up to places or be around certain people without one of your old disguises to hide behind, then it might be time to cut the strings.

Time is one of the most valuable assets you have in life, so in order to prioritize your own well-being and self-care, it will become necessary to say 'no' to certain situations or expectations. I know, even the thought of saying 'no' can present a real challenge for some, but this once again tends to be based on that fear of judgment from others. We fear saying 'no' for the reason that we fear upsetting someone or disappointing someone.

In reality, who is asking whom to be selfish? The three Cs—Context, Common sense and Confidence—will be your greatest friends here. Approaching these situations as your true-self will mean you are able to judge the situations presented to you from a logical mindset as opposed to emotional—and it was the fear that previously caused you to automatically say 'yes' to everything.

**Context:** *the circumstances that form the setting for an event, statement or idea, and in terms of which it can be fully understood.* So for example, your friend asks you to cancel your hair appointment and give her a lift into town. If she absolutely has to get to town for an interview, a bank meeting or a doctor's appointment, then it may be the sign of a good friend if you help her out. However, if she just wants to go shopping or is meeting another friend for coffee, then is it right for her to ask that you bypass your plans so that she can get to hers?

**Common sense:** *good sense and sound judgment in practical matters.* Take that same situation again, only this time you aren't doing anything special, perhaps just watching Netflix. You know that you could do with going into town also as you need some things, so common sense may prevail here as you understand that to do her this favor will not only not put you out, but it may also help you get some things done for yourself.

**Confidence:** *the feeling or belief that one can have faith in or rely on someone or something.* Remember, this is about relying on yourself to make a call on what *you* need. Work on building the confidence to put your needs first and say, "I'm so sorry, I can't—I already have plans."

That is just one example, but don't forget that even if you don't have plans per se, if you had just really been looking forward to chilling out in front of Netflix and know that you'd benefit from a rest, it's important to recognize that as being a good enough reason to say 'no.'

The kind of situations that this setting-boundaries task can include could be:

- Commitments/new projects/dates that you have no interest in attending
- Allowing people to walk all over you because of your fear of upsetting them
- Showing up to situations because you feel you 'should' rather than from a true desire to go
- Wasting your energy on lost causes

- Being in situations, or around certain people, that make you fearful of showing up as your true-self
- Being overlooked for important decisions or ideas because you are too fearful of putting your views across.

Why can't we do it all? Because at one point in the future, if not right now, it will get out of hand. Setting your own boundaries now, even if it means you use them to say 'yes' more, is fine as long as you are doing so while prioritizing your own well-being.

I want you to think back to the periods in your life when you have felt tired, burnt-out and drained—in this day and age, it's not uncommon for some of us to feel this most weeks. Often we blame the kids, our jobs, our friends or the housework, but these aren't really at the center of the problem. At the center of the issue lies our decision-making process. What is really to blame for being in this constant state of "I'm so tired" is our self-defeating habit of constantly saying 'yes' when we really mean 'no.'

Every day, colleagues, institutions, bosses, friends and family want you to attend to their needs. They don't do this because they are bad or selfish. They do this because it is simply what people do; they have their own best interests at heart. And you are also entitled to have your best interests at heart. You don't have to do what everyone else in society is doing. You are a unique combination of DNA, environment, culture and personal experiences. For you to say yes to something, it has to be special to you. Everything else, no matter what the consequences, you are entitled to say 'no' to.
—John Parkin, founder of the F**k It Life

We have become exceptionally good at accepting 'no' from others, but really bad at saying it. A lose-lose situation, really, huh? When someone else says 'no' to you, do you immediately think badly of them? Do you write them off as selfish and never to be trusted again? Again, this will (or should) depend on context. Have you ever felt grateful for someone saying 'no' to you? Saying 'no' also honors the fact that they know you deserve to have someone show up 100% in what you are asking. Being honest, putting your hands up and saying, "I'm just not in a position to give it what it deserves right now, but thank you for thinking of me," will not only show that you are in charge of your own life and mind, but it'll give you more space for what you *do* want to do. When you are asked to do something that truly gets your heart singing, you can grab it with both hands and graciously accept the offer without fear that you have taken on 'too much.'

Saying 'no' when you mean 'no' will open your life up to a whole lot more 'yes' experiences, without having the effect of exhaustion. You can show up to the things that grab your attention for the right reasons and spend your time with those who honor and respect your true-self without judgment. Learning the ability to say 'no' can be a powerful thing, just as powerful as learning when to say YES!

Say YES to the things that make your heart smile.

Say YES to following your gut instinct.

Say YES to things that you know will serve your highest good.

Say YES to things that fill you with energy.

Say YES to things you enjoy.

Say YES to feeling good!

# 34

# The Social Media Cull

The big S.M.! We have talked about this topic a bit earlier in the book, but not in an action-based, personalized way. So let me ask you this: what does real motivation look like to you? In the first part of this book, we talked a lot about the smoke and mirrors of the diet and fitness industries, including the 'fitspiration' trend that doesn't inspire but shames, the gurus who lead us on based on nothing but charmed looks and truth fabrication, and, of course, the highlighted news-reels of Facebook that have us questioning our every move.

Perhaps you now have accepted that the things that you may once have convinced yourself were motivating you to do, or be, better, were in fact acting as part of the problem, why you feel so down on yourself in the first place.

Protecting yourself from being dragged back into that negative, comparison-based mindset begins with you having a full social media blitz. Once your self-esteem is building and you are confident that you can show unconditional love and acceptance towards yourself, you may feel that you want to bring back whoever you decide to cull. However, I do suspect that when you have got to that point, you certainly won't feel the need to follow anyone that could potentially take you away from it!

First, it's about time to get really honest with yourself. Think carefully about who is in your life, social media or otherwise, that consistently makes you feel down on yourself or that you need to change who you are in order to be worthy of acceptance. Now, the key is to look in the places that you wouldn't immediately expect. The majority of clients I have done this with have still had the belief that the fitness and 'guru' pages that they follow are there purely to motivate and provide positive influence, but as we go over the criteria for positive influence versus shaming influence, it becomes clear to see that they are having a different effect than was thought. So let's take a look at those criteria:

Does the image/person/advice in question make you feel:

- Flawed?
- Bad?
- Defective?
- Not good enough?
- Unable to attain the 'ideal' results?
- Morally inferior?

You have to get really honest here, because you may be so used to feeling these emotions when looking at your social media pages that you actually struggle to identify what causes them and what doesn't.

So, let's move to the other side of the spectrum and do the other test; does it make you feel:

- Confident?
- Worthy?
- Positive?
- Does it leave you with a sense of self-acceptance?
- Does it make you feel good?
- Does it enhance your feelings of connection?

I want you to have this checklist in your mind the next time you scroll down your Facebook, Twitter or Instagram feeds. You can do this slowly but surely—you don't need to do it all at once, just as they come up. Each time you answer more 'yes's to the first list than to the second list, click the unfollow button.

You can tell when you are on the right path here as your daily social media sessions will shift from leaving you with a sense of shame and worthlessness to leaving you with a sense of positivity, love and worthiness.

*A quick note to end this section on: It is not a good idea to have to rely on others to keep you in check with these new positive feelings. Eventually, you will be able to feel secure in your sense of worthiness even when confronted by these pages or people you choose to unfollow. Your self-love will become impenetrable. Still, this culling is a temporary measure that will aid you in the process of making this full transition.*

# Attitude of Gratitude

Sonja Lyubomirsky, a positive psychologist from the University of California, Riverside, successfully demonstrated through scientific research that gratitude can increase the likelihood of a person becoming happier. There is a growing body of research out there that agrees with her. A simple but consistent practice of writing down three things you are grateful for every day significantly impacts our sense of appreciation, positivity and satisfaction.

This is going to form our next task. I want you to begin each morning or finish each night by writing down three things in your life that you feel gratitude for. This can be written in your journal before or after you do your meditation or it can be tapped in as a note in your phone as you walk to work—it doesn't need to take up much time, but the intention behind it is to stop for one moment and really think about those things that you feel grateful for.

Alongside understanding and appreciating the difference an attitude of gratitude can have, it's also important to recognize that to be grateful *doesn't* mean you can't pursue change. Being grateful can sometimes be mixed up with feelings such as "Well, I should just be happy with what I have." If you take out the word 'just,' then yes, this is correct. But there is no 'just' needed in this statement. 'Just' is a limiting word and it pushes the statement from gratitude-based to fear-based. Staying grateful in the moment for what you have does not mean you have to stop yourself from wanting to progress and make changes in your life. It is extremely difficult to be grateful and in a state of fear at the same time. Gratefulness will only be enhanced as you let yourself shift and move yourself towards living life authentically as your true-self.

As we discussed in Part One, it's often this lack of day-to-day fulfillment that leads us to that obsession with physical change, because it's that one area of our life (that we'd associated with increased feelings of happiness) that we still have a chance to change. Many people see being slimmer as their last chance of experiencing this fulfillment that society and the should-would-could pattern of their life has left them without. It's why it gets so frustrating for people when it doesn't happen. When that weight loss doesn't magically appear with total fulfillment as a side effect, the realization ensues that there is only one thing that will truly bring that—living a life without the masks. Spending every day as your true self, building your life around who you *are*, not who you think you should be.

There is a morning mantra spoken by the Dalai Lama that you may find helpful to recite quietly each time you are struggling to get into the mood for writing your grateful list. Those days will happen—but ironically, it's on those 'down' days that this process will help you the most!

Today I am fortunate to have woken up.
I am alive, I have a precious human life.
I am not going to waste it,
I am going to use all my energies to develop myself.
To expand my heart out to others,
To achieve enlightenment for the benefit of all beings.
I am going to have kind thoughts towards others,
I am not going to get angry or think badly about others,
I am going to benefit others as much as I can.

# 36

# Critical Thinking

I feel this will play an integral part in your escape from the clutches of the dieting industry, while still maintaining the ability to trust in the help that good coaches out there have to offer you.

Don't forget, I am not suggesting that you never wish to drop any weight ever again. I am simply enabling you to do so from a logical need, rather than an emotional one. In the future, you may feel like you wish to enlist the help of a coach and this will serve to give you far more power in your hunt for the right coach.

Critical thinking basically means thinking things through before making decisions or coming to conclusions. It's not getting drawn in by outrageous promises or caught up in all of the sales processes and tactics. There are a few vital questions to be asking yourself and the coach before you commit to giving away your time or money to this industry in the future. This brief list was put together by myself and a group of coaches in Richard Sennewald's online group membership site called 'Carbophobes.' As Richard explained earlier on, he prides himself on leaving a student with an ability to form opinions without bias as well as having the ability to understand and decipher critical information.

His teaching techniques are unique as he actively encourages students and clients to be open to changing their minds, leaving no room for conformation bias and always accepting the possibility that things aren't as black-and-white as they at first may seem.

Inquire as to what dietary approach they use; if they immediately reply with a 'label' such as Paleo, vegan, high-carb, etc., then an amber light should appear. The only really acceptable answer here would be "It depends." To give out dietary advice without first knowing everything about you, your lifestyle and your body can be a sign of a coach with set dogmas and paradigms.

Ask the coach what, if any, changes they have made to their approach in the last year and why. Most coaches will have made at least a few tweaks to what they advise and how they work. As we discussed, the science moves so fast, it's almost impossible to keep up, so it's not necessarily a bad thing if they have, but just be sure that they know why, so you know that they aren't just blindly following the industry trends.

At your first meeting with a coach, your questions to her are as important as hers are to you. You have every right to ask them what you need to know, too. If you feel uncomfortable in doing so, or if they don't seem very receptive to you asking, then again, this should be an amber light warning sign.

Ask for references for a few people they have worked with and if you could speak to them.

One last thing to remember: you should only be told what to eat specifically by a registered dietician. Any other coach—nutrition or otherwise—is not legally allowed to write individual meal plans.

If you visit any more than two of the above topics and feel uneasy about their answers, then go and find a few more coaches to visit first. By now, and certainly by the time you get to the end of this book and have been doing the mindset work for a few months, you will be on point and ready to go into any situation with a higher level of confidence than you had previously and this will help you in these kinds of situations. No longer will you ever need to feel indebted or grateful to a coach just for working with you and you should certainly never feel subservient ever again. If both parties are in it for the right reason, the relationship between coach and client can be a powerful one—founded on an equal, mutual standing.

While we are on the critical thinking topic, I feel it necessary to just briefly talk about the amazing, and barely understood, placebo effect. I expect you have heard of this at some time or another. It's important that you understand what this effect is, because unknowingly to most, it does have a place within the dieting industry. Let me explain how this could affect you.

**Placebo effect (also called the placebo response):** *A remarkable phenomenon in which a placebo—a fake treatment, an inactive substance like sugar, distilled water or saline solution—can sometimes improve a patient's condition simply because the person has the expectation that it will be helpful.*

The power of the mind is extraordinary and, in my opinion, it doesn't get even a tiny portion of the limelight that it deserves to in the field of health and well-being.

You'll likely have heard about this in articles when they cite the trials that medications have been put through to ensure their effectiveness, but when measuring the response to a placebo (a fake), they still see a response that they would expect from the *real* medicine on trial.

Where does this fit in with us? Well, it can work with food too. In certain circumstances, to expect to feel better on a certain restrictive diet can result in you experiencing that outcome, simply from the power of your expectation.

The following quote explains just how important this power of expectation can be:

Expectations appear to have a lot to do with the effect. If an intervention is believed to help a condition, a certain percentage of people who receive it will experience some benefit. How large a percentage varies tremendously and depends on the condition, the strength of belief, the subjectivity of the response and many other factors. The placebo effect may also have an element of psychological conditioning:

once someone benefits from an intervention, the person starts to associate that intervention with a benefit. The association, and therefore the benefit, may get stronger with additional exposures to the intervention.

—*Harvard Health Publications*, Harvard Medical School, 1 April 2012

I believe that this happens a lot with food and diets. Especially so now, when we seem to have so many practitioners who promote an idea that the more you cut out, the better and healthier a diet is. I've seen this industry trend pendulum swing all kinds of ways and it happens almost every time. Think back to when we all feared fat, all those years ago when saturated fat was the devil and we lived in fear of egg yolks. During that time, I recall talking to clients who were über-keen to promote their fat-free diet to others and they'd talk about how good they felt since going fat-free, leading the world to believe that a diet high in carbohydrates and grains was now the key to long-lasting health and abundant energy. And people thrived, they felt better, they felt energized—they felt what they *thought* they were supposed to feel.

Fast forward to the current trend and we've taken a turn to the complete opposite. We now live with a fear of carbs, resulting in a newfound appreciation for fat. So much so that I now hear on a regular basis how eating carbohydrates automatically leads people to a feeling of 'sleepiness' or lack of energy.

This certainly doesn't fit when we think about the energy levels of those who lived in the generations gone by (miners, factory workers, engineers) who worked exceedingly long days in far more physically rigorous roles than we see today, while enjoying their staple carbohydrate-based foods such as bread and jam.

I have no doubt that we have a new epidemic of those who feel unable to deal with carbohydrates, feeling sleepy after even looking at a bowl of oats, but I often wonder if this isn't also something to do with the expectation of feeling sleepy.

When we become aware that a majority of the popular Paleo bloggers are out there telling people that this is an expected side effect of eating carbs, we have to understand that these comments are likely to result in the expectation that this will happen. This is why I feel so strongly about nutrition coaches and health practitioners not promoting certain dietary methods or protocol publicly. Even witnessing a small, brief example of how a coach eats can implant a version of what is 'good' and 'bad' into a client's mind.

A nutrition plan should be individual, tailored around a client's adherence, preference and genuine medical history. In my opinion, the stress that comes with eliminating so many foods—alongside this expectation of physical reactions to certain ones—can cause much more harm than we realize.

So from here on in, by all means if you throw up every single time you eat bacon, then yes, it may be best to avoid it. If you've always gotten awful headaches each time you drink coffee, then avoid it. I wish that when I said "Use your common sense" it would be effective, but, without offending, I sometimes wonder whether the majority of our common sense has been all but scared out of us by the gurus. But I'll say it anyway. Listen to your body... and listen to your body *before* you take anything about bad food, sleepiness or 'toxins' as gospel.

Eat well! Not 'good' or 'bad,' just well.

# 37

# Embracing Your True-Self

*Waking up to who you are requires letting go of who you imagined yourself to be.*
— Alan Watts

You understand now what your true-self refers to and you have already started to peel back the layers of disguise to get to know your true-self, so here I want to combine what we have already found out from this journey so far with a little more digging, to help you to continue this true-self-discovery path. This section combines well with the previous one where we started to uncover your Self-Limiting Beliefs.

I left these final questions until now to give your previous work here a chance to sink in. So let's just go a bit further now.

Grab your journal again and start by pondering this question: What parts of my character did I feel I had to hide away in my childhood?

If you can recall that you always felt the need to hide a certain part of yourself in order to be who you thought you 'should' be, it can help you to understand where these fears of being seen as yourself originally stemmed from.

How did this change over the years?

What parts of my character did I feel I had to hide away in my teens?

What parts of my character did I feel I had to hide away yesterday?

Now we look back over the work you did earlier on with your self-limiting beliefs, this time coming at them from another angle as you start to make the connections.

> Do these character traits that I have spent my life trying to hide match up with the journaling questions I answered earlier on?

> Did my previously worn disguises cover up these aspects of me?

Understand that the real you, underneath all of the past efforts to 'cover up,' is worthy of love and acceptance, *always*.

These parts of you that you have tried to crush are often the most creative, passionate and unique parts of your character. To suppress yourself like this forever could mean that you never get to fully appreciate what these parts of you could do to enhance your life. Instead, we squash these 'non-conforming' parts of us down and try to be like everyone else. We choose to hide that part of us because we feel that it's not worth the risk of being judged, but all it does is leave us with a deep sense of emptiness and unfulfillment.

Embrace the times when you feel confident, secure and peaceful—you are showing up as your true-self.

Challenge the times that you feel any doubt, fear or uncertainty about yourself. You have two choices in these situations: you can either choose to take the risk of keeping your disguise off, stepping up and showing the world who you are—in essence, taking that risk of judgment—or you can simply choose to walk away from the situation.

Let your intuition guide you; it knows more than you think. If you are in a situation where you know that your true-self will not be accepted, maybe you genuinely fear that you will be harshly judged or ridiculed for showing who you are. If so, then please use everything you have learnt to dig deep and find the confidence to walk away.

The last task in this true-self quest is to invest in yourself more. Take time out, step away from everything, just for a day or even a few hours. Spend a day with yourself, with no demands on your time, no pressures to go or be anywhere. Many people say to me here, "What about a spa day?" Now, spa days are great, so if they make your heart sing and you get that genuine feeling of excitement in your gut about them, then absolutely — use them.

Still, I sometimes have to remind people that we are looking for a situation where you feel 100% comfortable being seen as you, no disguises, in all your rawness. So for many at this early stage, I have found that keeping it simple helps. Even just spending a day at home, but with no chores, absolutely no social media, no phone calls and no TV. Just you pottering around, reading, meditating and simply resting.

So many of us live in a constant state of 'doing' that the thought of switching off for a full day makes us recoil in horror. But allowing yourself to have a 'Me day' every few months can be akin to the purpose of giving your home a deep clean every so often. Once you do this deep clean "all-day-er," you know that it's just a case of topping yourself up with bite-sized chunks as and when you can for the next few months, which makes it a lot easier to achieve! This full day free can recharge your batteries faster and more effectively than six or seven choppy attempts where you try to allocate a few hours here or there.

If this suggestion of a day of rest sees your hackles rise from a deep-rooted fear of having a day of rest arise within you, then, as usual, this reaction can tell us something. We are so used to being busy that even when we are not, we choose to wear a disguise of 'busyness' that protects us from a fear of being judged. But what do you risk by taking a day of rest? A fear of being seen as lazy, unimportant or irrelevant? Where is the fear stemming from?

So just take a moment to go back and revisit the self-limiting belief questions with this before you go any further.

This may be the first time you will have given yourself permission to just 'be' for a while. Your mind may be on overdrive about all the things you need to get done and everything on your to-do list and how other people are relying on you. But the focus and reasoning for this day is to get to spend some time with yourself. If you cannot get even one day a year to spend on yourself, go back and revisit the Setting Boundaries section. In fact, re-read the entire second and third section — because remember, everything we are doing here has an underlying goal of you being able to live your life *for* you *as* you. Take your time with it. There really is no rush. Go back through all the journaling questions and really let yourself go deep where you need to.

Once you embark on this Me Day, if you struggle to switch off, it would be a great time to try a simple meditation. Personally, I found meditation to be absolutely integral to my journey towards self-acceptance, but I understand it's not for everyone. Again, if you find that it isn't a match for you, then don't force it. The idea behind it is to give your mind a chance to be still, to take a break from all those old scripts running through your mind and to help aid the process of planting your new beliefs (that you will be repeating every day). However, if you find that you are uncomfortable in practicing meditation, then perhaps try a walk among nature or a relaxing bath instead — anything that will see your mind calm and open to receiving these new thoughts.

A quick by the way on meditation: there are so many benefits to this practice, I would really recommend that you do try to include this in your daily life. There have been vast amounts of studies done since the practice became more popular in the Western world. It has been shown to decrease anxiety, depression and stress, reduce inflammation and increase positive emotion. So, for the purpose of this journey, I feel it will be an extremely beneficial addition. You needn't spend more than ten minutes a day on it; a simple 5–10 minutes in the morning can see you reaping these benefits.

Here is where many people let the familiar script of "I haven't got time!" rule their decision on whether or not this is possible, so here I challenge you to challenge this thought. Is this an old belief that you need to go back to and work on?

Is it absolutely true?

Let me put this to you a different way. If I said to you that I had a miracle drink that makes you happier, more fulfilled and more confident, but that you had to drink it slowly over ten minutes each morning, would you make the time to drink it? Oh, I expect you would! Time is all about priorities. You make time for the things you want to do. Don't fall into the quick-fix trap again—remember, you will reap these benefits long-term from all this shifting we are doing. That five-minute meditation is a part of that shift.

# 38

# Practicing Good Self-Care

This is the only section in the whole book where I am even going to mention nutrition, and even then, you'll see there are no prescription meal plans in sight. You know now that you don't need them. As I explained in detail over the course of Part One, there is only one thing we are absolutely certain of in the field of nutrition, and that is that there are no certainties.

The whole purpose of this process has been designed to help you realize that your confidence and self-esteem—therefore body image—is determined much more by how you *feel* than by how you look. It is also to help you to gain enough confidence in yourself and your abilities to escape from the shackles of the yo-yo diet culture, choosing to prioritize life, health, well-being and joy instead.

There really are only a few specifics in nutrition that I'd suggest always need to be adhered to when looking after your own well-being, so here is a very brief, basic list to work towards:

Eat a variety of colors and include a piece of fruit or plenty of veggies at every meal. Pack your meals with veggies to get them in without having to spend your time chained to a chopping board. I totally advocate the use of frozen veg for those who aren't confident in the kitchen purely for the simplicity and convenience. Whether you are making an omelet, a stir-fry or a pan of chili con carne, you can utilize frozen vegetables as you literally just have to chuck them into the pan and cook with the rest of the food.

Don't be afraid of fruits! All fruit is nutritious, but still contains calories so don't get caught in the trap of seeing fruit as a free-for-all. It's important to recognize that it's not sensible to graze on *any* food all day long, including fruit. In the great scheme of things, worrying about the sugar content of fruits isn't necessary unless the rest of your diet is sugar-packed. So eating fruit is a perfect time for you to practice the novel idea of context. Had a real carb-heavy day today? Probably choose some berries over a banana. But if you've feasted on mainly fats and proteins, then a banana split can be a lovely (and delicious) addition to your day.

Ensure you are drinking enough water, but you don't need to chug it down all day every day; there is no need to overthink this but just simply get used to reaching for a glass of water a few times a day. If you drink tons and tons of coffee or tea then perhaps swap one or two for a glass of water and see how you feel. If you sweat more, drink more—keep it simple.

Ensure you are getting enough protein—aim for a fist-sized portion at most meals. Protein shakes are great for convenience again and if you like milkshakes then protein smoothies could be a great thing to implement to kill two birds with one stone. Again, don't overthink this! If you miss out a source of protein one meal nothing scary will happen; you will not immediately start to shrivel up and turn to mush. Just have a portion at your next meal.

Utilize the 85% rule as best you can. Begin to see food a little like you would your bank balance: if you spent a bit more on a pair of shoes last week, naturally you don't go out and buy another expensive pair this week. You manage it. You view it with logic. You certainly don't burst into tears, prod the shoes and complain that they've ruined everything and that you now have to live on coupons for the rest of the month.

Moderation and flexibility are not sexy; we know this and this is why it doesn't sell. But let me tell you a secret: between total and utter life-controlling restriction (aka 'orthorexia') and binge, binge, binge eat ALL the food, lies a huge, vast gray area called *balance*. Living, and eating, with balance means that you *can* eat 85% 'natural' and wholesome foods in the week but still enjoy a fresh-bread bacon buttie with ketchup on a Sunday morning.

If you struggle to maintain that flexibility without it leading to a binge, then it's time to recognize that potentially food itself isn't the problem, but your behavior around food is, and it's imperative to understand that there is a huge difference between the two.

As I'm writing this I'm trying to resist the temptation to make it more complicated, to include some "shocking hints" that will really grab your attention, but that will defeat the entire purpose of this book. The diet industry has massively overcomplicated nutrition to the point where grown adults are now often to be found quivering and panicking at buffet tables as they try to decide what to have that 'fits' with whatever plan it is they are on. It has made coaches nervous about recommending this age-old idea of balance and flexibility because it's now seen as not radical enough.

Believe me, once we find that one-size-fits-all, single, proven way to eat for health, well-being and longevity, we'll surely all know about it. But for now, we haven't—and don't let anyone try to convince you otherwise. We haven't, we really haven't. So until then let's just cap the hysteria and regain a little of that lost common sense when it comes to choosing what to eat.

And lastly, don't cut out any whole food groups, unless you have had specific, individual advice from a qualified GP or dietician.

Eat carbs, eat fats, eat a bit of what you fancy every now and then, and most importantly, view everything in context.

You are smarter than you think when it comes to your own body and it's time to trust yourself a bit more.

A hugely important thing to recognize is this: you can have the most expensive, detailed, tailored nutrition plan in the whole world, but it will be absolutely and utterly useless if you don't enjoy and can't adhere to it.

A *good* diet is the one that you can follow without stress, without having to miss out on social occasions, and one that you enjoy, forever.

A *successful* diet plan is the one that you are still following ten years down the line, having maintained a healthy weight consistently for the majority of that time.

The easiest way to ensure this? Back to the balance and flexibility card. There is a likelihood that you may be unsure how to go about getting some balance and flexibility back into your diet if you have been following strict rules or have been told to cut a gazillion things out, so if you are at a point where you have become fearful about adding certain foods back into your diet then please, seek help.

Remember that food doesn't have morals. No food is inherently good, or bad—the devil is always in the dosage. If you eat a doughnut, you are not 'naughty,' and it wasn't 'bad.' You just ate a doughnut. Take away the connection of what you eat to who you are. Next time you go a little overboard with the cheese board, simply state the situation as it is: "Oh shucks, I went a little too heavy with the cheese board there!" But you are not a bad person for doing so, so take away the "I am..." And replace it with "I did..."

If you are constantly struggling with excess weight and if you are holding enough to mean that your health is suffering as a result, then I would always suggest trying to find out the most suitable (tailored for you) and balanced way in which you are able to get this under control, but please do so under the guidance of professional help.

As mentioned earlier on, I am absolutely not against dieting, but I feel it's hugely important to separate the need for health-related dieting as far away as possible from self-esteem and confidence-related appearance-fixing. Remember, you eat well to take care of your body, *not* to increase your sense of worthiness as a person.

If it becomes clear during this process that the reason for this excess weight is emotionally led (binge eating, emotional eating, any type of disordered eating), I wouldn't recommend that you only try to deal with this yourself; be brave enough and honor yourself by seeking some help. Go visit someone who offers specialized therapy, a psychologist, psychiatrist or eating disorder specialist. Once again, it's often not what you are eating, but why you are eating it that is causing the struggles behind a person's long-term weight battles. No diet plan will help that— no matter how balanced and flexible it is. You need to dig deeper into the emotional reasons behind your struggles, and by doing so, there needn't be any shame associated, only bravery. To sum this up:

- Eat a variety of colors—include a piece of fruit or plenty of veggies at most meals.
- Ensure you are drinking enough water. You don't need to chug it down all day every day, just get used to reaching for a glass of water a few times a day as a replacement for a coffee or two. If you sweat more, drink more!
- Ensure you are getting enough protein, aiming for a fist-sized portion at most meals.
- Don't cut out any whole food groups, unless you have had specific, individual advice from a qualified GP or dietician.
- Remember and respect that calories are still king when it comes to weight gain, loss or maintenance.
- Eat a bit of what you fancy now and then.
- View everything in CONTEXT.

You are smarter than you think when it comes to your own body. Start to take more notice of your intuition and trust yourself to believe what your own body is telling you.

## 39

# Putting the Love into Self-Love

We are nearing the end of this journey. I hope that by this point you are feeling a huge increase in the amount of love and acceptance that you have for yourself. Self-love is much harder to achieve than self-hate. We have had a lot of practice with the latter and hardly any with the former! But you are now at the start of a whole new path which is leading you towards a life where you can wake up each and every day with that inherent knowing that you are 'enough,' no matter what. No longer will you have the underlying emotion of worthlessness; no longer will you need to wear a different disguise in every situation in order to feel accepted. You will gain energy from not having to censor, pretend or promote yourself to feel worthy, you will gain vitality as you begin to open up to and appreciate those in your life who love you for who you are, while stepping back from those who don't, and you will begin to wonder why you spent so long accepting life within this false-self prison!

Self-love and acceptance is a freedom; it's an opportunity to go forth and live your life as you, offering the world an opportunity to see who you are at your core as you go forth and seek out your places of joy. The relief you feel as the fear and disguises begin to fall away will be mixed with anxiety at first, but remember, that vulnerability that you have to lean into in order to be able to do this will present to you opportunities to grow real bonds and make lasting connections with those around you who truly count. As this happens, you will notice how this very experience of being loved and accepted for your true-self will only serve to build and contribute towards the growth of love for yourself.

You will have bad days. Heck, we all have them. Self-love isn't about reaching cloud-nine levels of self-appreciation every single day for the rest of your life, because there will be times when you want to kick yourself, when you look in the mirror and don't feel completely in love with what you see, but the goal we are aiming for is consistency.

The end of this book signifies the end of my part in your journey, but by no means does this mean that your journey is done. This is only just the beginning for you. Make everything you have learnt here a habit, invest the time in yourself, spend time with the journaling questions and go back and revisit the tasks. Just keep going. This is your big, lifetime opportunity to start over and to finally let go of all the constraining beliefs about who you think you are supposed to be.

# Values List

| | |
|---|---|
| Abundance | Assurance |
| Acceptance | Attentiveness |
| Accessibility | Attractiveness |
| Accomplishment | Audacity |
| Accountability | Availability |
| Accuracy | Awareness |
| Achievement | Awe |
| Acknowledgment | Balance |
| Activeness | Beauty |
| Adaptability | Being the best |
| Adoration | Belonging |
| Adroitness | Benevolence |
| Advancement | Bliss |
| Adventure | Boldness |
| Affection | Bravery |
| Affluence | Brilliance |
| Aggressiveness | Buoyancy |
| Agility | Calmness |
| Alertness | Camaraderie |
| Altruism | Candor |
| Amazement | Capability |
| Ambition | Care |
| Amusement | Carefulness |
| Anticipation | Celebrity |
| Appreciation | Certainty |
| Approachability | Challenge |
| Approval | Change |
| Art | Charity |
| Articulacy | Charm |
| Artistry | Chastity |
| Assertiveness | Cheerfulness |

Clarity

Cleanliness

Clear-mindedness

Cleverness

Closeness

Comfort

Commitment

Community

Compassion

Competence

Competition

Completion

Composure

Concentration

Confidence

Conformity

Congruency

Connection

Consciousness

Conservation

Consistency

Contentment

Continuity

Contribution

Control

Conviction

Conviviality

Coolness

Cooperation

Cordiality

Correctness

Country

Courage

Courtesy

Craftiness

Creativity

Credibility

Cunning

Curiosity

Daring

Decisiveness

Decorum

Deference

Delight

Dependability

Depth

Desire

Determination

Devotion

Devoutness

Dexterity

Dignity

Diligence

Direction

Directness

Discipline

Discovery

Discretion

Diversity

Dominance

Dreaming

Drive

Duty

Dynamism

Eagerness

Ease

Economy

Ecstasy

Education

Effectiveness

Efficiency

Elation

Elegance

Empathy

Encouragement

Endurance

Energy

Enjoyment

Entertainment

Enthusiasm

Environmentalism

Ethics

Euphoria

Excellence

Excitement

Exhilaration

Expectancy

Expediency

Experience

Expertise

Exploration

Expressiveness

Extravagance

Extroversion

Exuberance

Fairness

Faith

Fame

Family

Fascination

Fashion

Fearlessness

Ferocity

Fidelity

Fierceness

Financial independence

Firmness

Fitness

Flexibility

Flow

Fluency

Focus

Fortitude

Frankness

Freedom

Friendliness

Friendship

Frugality

Fun

Gallantry

Generosity

Gentility

Giving

Grace

Gratitude

Gregariousness

Growth

Guidance

Happiness

Harmony

Health

Heart

Helpfulness

Heroism

Holiness

Honesty

| | |
|---|---|
| Honor | Kindness |
| Hopefulness | Knowledge |
| Hospitality | Leadership |
| Humility | Learning |
| Humor | Liberation |
| Hygiene | Liberty |
| Imagination | Lightness |
| Impact | Liveliness |
| Impartiality | Logic |
| Independence | Longevity |
| Individuality | Love |
| Industry | Loyalty |
| Influence | Majesty |
| Ingenuity | Making a difference |
| Inquisitiveness | Marriage |
| Insightfulness | Mastery |
| Inspiration | Maturity |
| Integrity | Meaning |
| Intellect | Meekness |
| Intelligence | Mellowness |
| Intensity | Meticulousness |
| Intimacy | Mindfulness |
| Intrepidness | Modesty |
| Introspection | Motivation |
| Introversion | Mysteriousness |
| Intuition | Nature |
| Intuitiveness | Neatness |
| Inventiveness | Nerve |
| Investing | Noncomformity |
| Involvement | Obedience |
| Joy | Open-mindedness |
| Judiciousness | Openness |
| Justice | Optimism |
| Keenness | Order |

Organization

Originality

Outdoors

Outlandishness

Outrageousness

Partnership

Patience

Passion

Peace

Perceptiveness

Perfection

Perkiness

Perseverance

Persistence

Persuasiveness

Philanthropy

Piety

Playfulness

Pleasantness

Pleasure

Poise

Polish

Popularity

Potency

Power

Practicality

Pragmatism

Precision

Preparedness

Presence

Pride

Privacy

Proactivity

Professionalism

Prosperity

Prudence

Punctuality

Purity

Rationality

Realism

Reason

Reasonableness

Recognition

Recreation

Refinement

Reflection

Relaxation

Reliability

Relief

Religiousness

Reputation

Resilience

Resolution

Resolve

Resourcefulness

Respect

Responsibility

Rest

Restraint

Reverence

Richness

Rigor

Sacredness

Sacrifice

Sagacity

Saintliness

Sanguinity

Satisfaction

Science

Security

Self-control

Selflessness

Self-reliance

Self-respect

Sensitivity

Sensuality

Serenity

Service

Sexiness

Sexuality

Sharing

Shrewdness

Significance

Silence

Silliness

Simplicity

Sincerity

Skillfulness

Solidarity

Solitude

Sophistication

Soundness

Speed

Spirit

Spirituality

Spontaneity

Spunk

Stability

Status

Stealth

Stillness

Strength

Structure

Success

Support

Supremacy

Surprise

Sympathy

Synergy

Teaching

Teamwork

Temperance

Thankfulness

Thoroughness

Thoughtfulness

Thrift

Tidiness

Timeliness

Traditionalism

Tranquillity

Transcendence

Trust

Trustworthiness

Truth

Understanding

Unflappability

Uniqueness

Unity

Usefulness

Utility

Valor

Variety

Victory

Vigor

Virtue

Vision

Vitality
Vivacity
Volunteering
Warm-heartedness
Warmth
Watchfulness
Wealth
Willfulness

Willingness
Winning
Wisdom
Wittiness
Wonder
Worthiness
Youthfulness
Zeal

# Epilogue

Since you are reading these concluding words and my parting thoughts to follow, I know you have already forged a commitment to embark on a new way of life. This is wonderful news to me, for which I offer you a heartfelt thank-you!

I've presented a lot of information to you throughout the book, and even if you haven't begun to actively engage with it, I know that you'll have the opportunity to pull bits out from your memory as and when you need it. Naturally, you can come back to any part of it at any time. I truly hope that our exploration together will bring a positive shift of some kind within you, and I will feel forever grateful for being able to play my part in making that shift possible.

I have hinted within the pages of this book about some of my not-so-good times but I want to make it very clear that I have absolutely no regrets about anything that I have experienced in my life or career because, quite frankly, if I hadn't done the things, felt the things, been around the things and seen the things that I have, then I wouldn't have written this book for you. I wouldn't be able to coach so powerfully had I not spent time on both sides of the fence and I certainly wouldn't ever have known the almighty impact that all of the issues contained in this book could have on a woman's perception of herself.

I have taken many, many risks within my working life in order to spread this message of self-love. I have done things that many would (and did) call me crazy for. One thing I have learned is that if you want something, you have to be prepared to take risks. This isn't just in work or career circumstances—it's an integral part of life. You have to risk losing something you *don't* want in order to gain something you *do* want.

I grew up with loving parents, in a loving home, with two brothers and a cat. There was nothing extraordinary about my upbringing, and yet, so many times, my mum has asked me "Where did all those insecurities come from?" To this day, I really don't know. My subconscious was exposed to, and took notice of, everything and anything that led me to question who I was and if *what* I was could ever be worthy enough. It starts to make a bit more sense when you look at the ideals I grew up with. My parents were total opposites—so when people say opposites attract, I can see why: fifty years of marriage later and still laughing together every day. My dad always encouraged me to go for my dreams. Whatever they were at the time, he encouraged me to follow them. I always remember he kept a list of affirmations in his desk about the things he wanted to do, achieve and become. He was always on the verge of a break-through in business, he had many set-backs and disappoint-ments, but one thing I always remember is that he always kept that belief of real possibility within him. My mum, however, was often to be found pulling her hair out in despair about the latest business idea or opportunity he'd come up with. She always did, and still does, value safety and security as something not ever to be risked.

That safety and security came, in her eyes, in the form of a steady 9-to-5 office job that she kept for nearly her entire working life. Change is not something my mum goes after and when it does present itself, she views it with caution and fear. Unsurprisingly, it may seem, as she lost her father suddenly and unexpectedly at the age of 17, that maybe as a consequence of this, she learned to view change as a negative experience.

As you can imagine, this conflict of teaching as I grew up created extreme ebbs and flows in my own ideas of what I wanted to do and what I believed I could achieve within my own life. I remember one day I found myself sitting behind the checkout of a supermarket, which delighted my mum no end, as to her this was conducive to a safe, secure and long-term plan of employment. But all I felt was trapped.

I remember my dad having a way with his words and he always managed to find a way to encourage me to take the risk and go for what I really wanted, but he did so in a manner that meant my mum had no way of detecting that he'd just encouraged me to quit my 'safe' job. We used to have secret chats where, even though the words weren't said, I knew he was giving me the nod of support to do whatever it was I was dreaming about doing.

So I have had the opportunity to see how different it could have been, had I been more like my mum. I think about where I would have ended up, where I would be now had I had two parents who both associated office work with 'real work' and security, who viewed, as many do, self-employed coaching as risky. Would I have still listened to that little voice within me, the one that has always been there telling me to go with my passion, telling me to follow this path and go for that opportunity, telling me that my dream of changing the world one person at a time wasn't impossible? Who knows?

Even so, I am grateful to both my mum and dad for being true to themselves. I also want to thank them for showing me possibly some of the greatest examples of differing mindsets and how they can completely and utterly change that person's view of a situation. Above all else, I want to thank them both for all the continued support—in both of their own unique, different ways—as I have absolutely no doubt that if it wasn't for their overriding trust and belief in me, my life would have turned out very different.

As I look back now over my epiphany-fueled burnout journey that led to the creation of this book, I am more and more convinced that this was brought on by a crisis of identity. I'd spent so long marking my territory as this super-disciplined coach who had frogmarched so many others into the elite 'health and well-being' camp of clean eating, grueling exercise and self-deprivation, yet now here I was suddenly having come to the realization that everything I'd been doing was having the opposite effect to how I truly wanted to live and feel.

Throughout this period, I was barely able to hold a conversation with a client without feeling overwhelmed and close to tears. All I wanted to do was give up, hide under my duvet and go back to being born so I could start this game of life all over again. I knew I was risking a lot by completely changing my stance on everything I'd once believed and encouraged. I had to effectively rebuild myself as a coach and it would have been so much easier to just carry on and pretend. I could have continued to do what I was doing. No one really even had to know that I'd had this mini-breakdown within my own mind. Still, I felt pulled, I felt compelled to share it; I felt it was only right to help those people who wanted to be told that it's really okay and acceptable to be themselves, that they aren't mad, crazy or lazy for not conforming to the perfect existence that the billboards depict.

Truth be told, the unrelenting frustration I felt during those days was nearly overwhelming, but because I was in such a dark hole, unable to climb out, I just couldn't see that I was perpetuating this cycle of feelings by continuing to do what I was doing. I'd be sitting there, feeling on the verge of total exhaustion from trying to recalibrate my life, but thinking that if I just 'hustled' a bit harder, spent a bit more time on social media, or worked a little bit longer that day, it would all go away and everything would be fixed. Only now do I know that it was those methods of thinking that were perpetuating the feelings I was trying to escape from.

As the great Einstein once said, "We can't solve problems by using the same kind of thinking we used when we created them."

Ironically, clarity is something that only comes to you when you allow yourself to accept the possibility that something you are doing currently isn't working. Clarity lives in those 'a-ha' light bulb realization moments, the moments when you sit on the stairs with your head in your hands and think *I just can't do this anymore.* Only then do you truly accept that there may be a different, easier way to get where it is that you are trying to go.

Whether you are thinking about your physical, emotional or mental health, change always has to begin with desire, a strong, true, burning sense of urgency that then is followed up by commitment.

In order to get out from this black hole and back into a place of peace, I knew that I had to change something about the way I was living. It meant I had to take risks—financial and personal—in order to create that change, but I knew what I wanted. I had a vision in my head of how I wanted my life to be and I chose to do what I had to do in order to create that life. Previously, this would have been a prime opportunity for me to have thrown my hands up into the air and quit. Because, believe me, there have been times when I have done just that. I could have easily just given up and gone out to find a steady job, away from the industry, and quit coaching, knowing that overnight all the stresses that came with it would disappear.

Still, I knew what I was trying to do and I knew the message that I was trying to spread was worth that risk. I just had to learn how to manage myself better. You see, the external situations weren't the problem; *I* was. I wasn't being forced to do anything. I made my own choices. Only I had the power to change the way I thought, which in turn changed the way I lived.

My burnout was a side effect of other, deeper issues that had been bubbling up ever since I started to care so much about the way I came across to other people. This desire to be seen as this honed, disciplined and faultless coach had leaked into every area of my life. Only when I managed to let go of that continual all-encompassing fear of judgment was I able to choose purpose-fully how I felt each day, about myself, my work and my life. In letting go of the control of how *others* viewed me, I was able to take back the control of my own life and my own happiness.

Ever since then, I have felt it was my turn to *return* this act of empowerment, to use all of my experience—personal and professional—and my coaching skills to aid other people in their escape from the prison within their own minds. To help you to release yourself from all the limiting beliefs that hold you back from a fear of being seen as, and being proud of, the person that you truly are. This is what I continue to do every day through my words written and spoken, and will do as long as I can. I truly hope that this is what I have been able to do for you.

Never again apologize for who you are, for you are greatness personified. Always live with this statement in your heart: *I am better than no one, yet no one is better than me.*

With love, power and awesomeness,
Heather

CHANGE
MAKERS
BOOKS

Changemakers publishes books for individuals committed to transforming their lives and transforming the world. Our readers seek to become positive, powerful agents of change. Changemakers books inform, inspire, and provide practical wisdom and skills to empower us to create the next chapter of humanity's future.
Please visit our website at www.changemakers-books.com